HOME REMEDIES

HYDROTHERAPY MASSAGE CHARCOAL AND OTHER SIMPLE TREATMENTS

For use in the home, and under field conditions by both laymen and
skilled medical persons.

by

Agatha Moody Thrash, M.D.

and

Calvin L. Thrash, Jr., M.D.

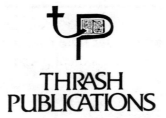

THRASH
PUBLICATIONS

Rt. 1, Box 273
Seale, Alabama 36875

ISBN: 0-942658-02-7

CREDITS

The work of many people goes into the making of a book. We should like to mention a few of those contributing especially generously toward HOME REMEDIES.

The art work was done by Alice Sarah Eisler and Cal Thrash. Editing was done by Marjorie Baldwin, M.D., Nelsy Restrepo, M.D., David Miller, M.D., and Martha Seeley, M.D., George Kendall, contributed his assistance in literary styling, and also called upon his extensive experience in hydrotherapy.

The authors would like to thank particularly their research librarian, Phylis Austin, for the large amount of library time required for such a project, for the preparation of bibliography and index, and the meticulous stenographic work. Thanks should also go to Lois Prest and Carol Sims. Cover concept by Dennis Davis.

Last, our thanks go to our children, Ann and Cal, for patiently submitting through the years, to experimentation in the home setting and to our students and patients who have taught us much. May those who use this book be blessed by their contributions.

The Authors

CONTENTS

PREFACE

Over the past fifteen years, we have seen an increasing interest in discovering and using methods of healing that would be simple, rational, effective, but yet would leave no ill effects on the patient. These methods have largely involved various physical therapy modalities, simple herb teas, dietotherapy, and cleanliness, both internal and external. They have included a variety of physiological stimuli to be used in a home setting under different circumstances of disease—inflammatory states, neoplasms, degenerative diseases, and mental illnesses.

Having been thoroughly schooled in the allopathic methods of treating disease used generally by M.D.'s, it was no small matter to make the changes in thinking necessary to accept as true remedies those treatments that call for few drugs and rely on the physiological processes that ultimately bring about all healing.

The healing process involves only the following known factors: blood and lymph vessels, nerve stimuli, leukocytes, connective tissue, plasma proteins, biochemical mechanisms, and immune properties of living cells. Therefore, it has become progressively more clear to us that it is only those remedies that assist, stimulate, remove impediments, and direct nature in her efforts to throw off an offending agent and utilize the defense mechanisms of the body that can be classed as true remedies.

When one accepts these widely known but poorly appreciated facts, it becomes obvious that almost anything that is done merely to alleviate symptoms cannot effect a cure, but actually interferes with the genuine healing processes of the body itself. In fact, these drastic methods usually poison some part of the defense mechanism. It also becomes immediately obvious that based on the need it senses, the body generally activates the mechanisms of healing it will be using to the utmost, being limited mainly by the inhibiting influences of poor foods, chilling, various chemicals including drugs, and a deleterious life style.

At the Medical College of Georgia, Dr. Phillip Dow taught for many years that normal physiological processes are basic to all healing, and that no method, drug, or procedure could substitute for the process. He taught that the best that can be done by any external influence is to take away toxic substances, keep the field clean, provide necessary raw materials, remove all interfering influences, and wait for the body to activate its marvelous recuperative resources.

At the same school Dr. Edgar Pund made certain that all his students in pathology understood that the equipment of the body is adequate to carry on needed processes of inflammation and repair, and that even pain and fever are protective and healing in their objectives. These physiologic responses to noxious agents should not be carelessly or needlessly subdued as they can be effective aids in the activation of defenses.

Caretaking in small details can turn the tide in the treatment of disease. All parts of the body and mind are interrelated. Even a discouraging attitude held by either the therapist or the patient can have a depressing influence on the outcome of a treatment. Every kind of unfavorable agent should be eliminated, for on a very small matter can rest success or failure in the treatment of disease. During the past ten years, it has been our rare privilege to put most of these techniques into effect at Yuchi Pines Institute, a medical missionary training school operated by Seventh-day Adventist laymen. Beset by inexperience and lack of knowledge, we began haltingly and timidly. Gradually confidence, skill, and experience have grown as the Lord blessed our efforts and strengthened our faith through remarkable improvements or cures in both the common diseases as well as rare and difficult cases.

Both by study and experience we began to understand something of the nature of the rational or physiologic remedies in the treatment of disease. We began to suspect that there were others in the medical profession using rational therapy whose experiences would assist us to treat disease with simple remedies. We began to search the medical literature for experiences of earlier physiotherapists. We were surprised to find an overwhelming number of examples that clearly pointed

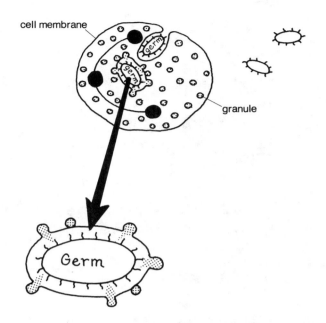

Germs imprisoned in a segment of cell membrane are brought inside the neutrophil. The cell can engulf several germs simultaneously in 5-10 minutes after encounter, a process called phagocytosis. Then the granules containing the powerful digestants migrate to the capsule containing the germ, join their own capsules into the membrane capsule surrounding the germ (note enlargement), pour the digestants in on the germ; death of the germ quickly occurs.

Neutrophils subsist almost entirely by glycolysis ("burning" sugars to lactic or pyruvic acid) rather than by respiration (complete oxidation to carbon dioxide and water). Neutrophils produce large quantities of lactic acid, especially after phagocytosis (feeding). Hydrogen peroxide, a good germicide, is produced by the oxidases of the granules. The granules also contain certain peptides. It thus appears that the neutrophil is equipped with a considerable "overkill" capacity. When a neutrophil engulfs material which it cannot digest (carbon, waxes, etc.) the cell may spit the material out or may carry it in its own body to the "graveyard" or the outside environment (intestine, breast, sweat glands or genitourinary secretions).

The Army Weakened

Migration of white blood cells and margination on blood vessel linings preparatory to entering the tissues for policing or in response to chemical attraction (chemotaxis) are both impaired by cortisone. Certain congenital abnormalities of neutrophils impair their function. Some such neutrophils lack the powerful digestive enzymes in the granules. Some granules are giant-sized

but unable to function well. Some of these abnormalities in white blood cells are associated with partial albinism. These abnormal granules cannot properly fuse with the capsules which contain germs as described above.[18] It is likely that prenatal influences have an effect on the development of the mechanism to produce proper blood cells. Many, if not most of these inborn abnormalities in white blood cells are the result of toxic injury from the repeated contacts with mutagens in our chemical environment. Pregnant women should be especially protected from all drugs and toxic chemicals. Drugs, both licit and illicit, caffeine, alcohol, and the infections which the mother suffers during as well as prior to pregnancy may all have an influence on the factors that determine these fine points of cellular development. An unborn baby may have the equipment for making white blood cells permanently damaged by drugs and chemicals the mother is exposed to during her pregnancy.

Human Leukocyte Antigens (HLA)

Human leukocyte antigens (HLA) have recently been discovered to have an association with human disease, particularly rheumatic disease. HLA tissue typing has been used for some time to try to match organ transplants. That the HLA's could be used in human disease is a fairly new thought. The sixth somatic chromosome carries the genes for immune responses. We began to understand something about HLA's in 1952 when patients receiving multiple blood transfusions were shown to agglutinate leukocytes. Similarly, after pregnancy, agglutinins to leukocytes are formed. The HLA system is the major histocompatibility complex in man enabling the cells to distinguish their *own relatives* from any *other human cells.*

In addition to HLA, the sixth chromosome is responsible for many serum proteins, several complement components, red cell antigens, immune response genes, and phosphoglucomutase. In other words, *the ability to* defend oneself against a germ *is inherited* through the sixth chromosome. A person expresses his antigens, which he receives from both mother and father, in a codominant fashion. Crossovers and deletions of chromosomes do occur giving opportunity for damage to the antigen-making areas by *maternal drug exposure, diet and poor health habits.* HLA's are special chemicals synthesized in the white blood cells and are composed of glycoproteins. They become attached to the exterior of the cell membranes, and are thereby exposed to all the extracellular environment. They are somewhat race specific. As an example, the Negro race has HLA Aw-19 in 54% of the population. In contrast, only 13% of Cauca-

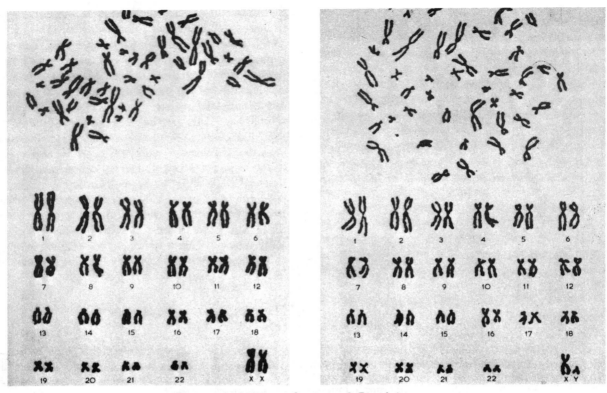

Elements of Human Anatomy & Physiology

Human karyotype. In the top of the figure the chromosomes are scattered as they grew in the dividing cell. Below they have been sorted and grouped in the 22 somatic (body) pairs and one sex pair. The cells are "caught" at this stage, photographed, and the photograph actually cut out to produce the chromosomes which are then pasted on a sheet that has 1-22 somatic pairs and a single sex pair in the lower right which determine maleness or femaleness. XX is female, Xy is male. A good quality chromosome pair in position #6 is necessary in order to produce perfect HLA (human leukocyte antigen) and many other serum proteins active in defense.

sians express Aw-19. Many antigens are inherited in a clone or cluster. It may be that through this mechanism the likelihood of developing diseases such as diabetes, multiple sclerosis, and rheumatoid arthritis is genetically controlled. This wonderful mechanism, so orderly in its minutest detail, is the wise and loving provision of the Master Designer. By carefully avoiding injury from drugs and disease we can pass down as a precious legacy these unspeakably valuable genetic treasures.

The sixth chromosome has at least four loci (positions on a chromosome) where antigens are determined. It has been shown that the "D" position carries the determinance for an antigen which will be concentrated on the cell membranes of bone marrow-derived lymphocytes, macrophages, monocytes, and endothelial cells, all cells capable of being stimulated by germs and inflammatory processes. These antigens which are on lymphocytes derived from bone marrow, occur with higher frequency in individuals who have multiple sclerosis or leukemias than in persons who do not have these disorders.

More Factors that Influence Healing

Many factors influence the development or location of an infection: 1) the number of white blood cells that are available to circulate in the blood stream during the emergency, 2) the rate of locomotion of the white blood cells, 3) the "interest" these cells have in "eating" germs, 4) their success in killing the germs taken in, 5) as well as other processes of local and general nature involving the blood vessels, 6) the immune system, 7) the general health, and many other factors. The rapidity with which the phagocytes, the "eating cells", travel to an infection, as well as the liberation of enzymes at the site of infection are prime defense mechanisms.

Heating the part which harbors an infection hastens the rate at which leukocytes move into the area and liberate their enzymes.[19] Van't Hoff's law states that the velocity of a chemical reaction is approximately doubled or tripled by a rise in temperature of 10°.

Wound healing time in the skin of alligators is shortened two to three times by a rise in temperature of 10 degrees. Ants move twice as rapidly at 21° as at 11° C.[20] It has been found that the rate of locomotion of leukocytes into an infected area determines the amount of phagocytosis (eating by cells) and liberation of enzymes that will be available to clear up the infection. The most rapid rate of locomotion occurs at 40° C. (104° F.), whereas there is a depression of locomotion at 42° C. (107.6°). Prognosis in infections therefore is usually *more favorable* if neither local nor systemic temperatures exceed 104°, but do rise four to five degrees above normal.[21] So effective is fever in helping fight infection and other inflammatory disorders that artificial fevers have been used extensively for disease treatment. Artificial fevers have been induced in the past by a number of methods, the most outstanding of which are the following: malaria inoculations, injection of foreign protein and other toxic substances, diathermy, high frequency electrostatic field and hydrotherapy (hot baths).[22]

In an extensive study of physiologic changes during and after artificial fever therapy, investigators found blood counts before and after five hours of sustained fever at 105° to 106° showed a rise in white blood cells circulating in the blood from 6,800 to 13,200, and average hemoglobin levels of 12.0 before and 11.8 afterward. The authors reported another study of 100 patients with a duration of artificial fever from three to seven hours at temperatures from 104° to 106.8° which showed leukocytes 7,125 and 11,269 before and after, with hemoglobin levels at 13.3 before and after.[23] It was believed that the bone marrow delivery of reserve mature white blood cells was the important feature here, and not a redistribution phenomenon of leukocytes from storage areas.

A study was done on the locomotion of white blood cells at different temperatures. The control group of 10 cells, all at 37° C. (98.6° F) traveled an average distance of 175 micra in five minutes. As the temperature of the white blood cells was taken up from 27° to 40° C. at least twice the rate of movement was observed in their locomotion at the higher temperatures. An increased rate of intracellular killing by lymphocytes is quite active at one hour[24] and probably persists two hours after the temperature has returned to normal.

Madsen and Wulff found that the optimum phagocytic index, the rate at which germs are engulfed by a white blood cell, corresponds closely with the normal temperature of the species from which the leukocytes were taken. In man, 37° C; in guinea pig 39° C; and in birds, 41° C., represented the optimum temperatures for phagocytosis to occur, each being the normal temperature

for that species. In the cold-blooded frog, phagocytosis was the same at all temperatures between 9° and 37° C.[25] This is no chance adaptation. It is evidence of the life sustaining power of God.

Rate of Locomotion of Leucocytes at Different Temperatures[26]

Temperature in Centigrade	Mean Distance Travelled in 5 minutes
23°	31.4 micra
27°	82.8 micra
33°	134.6 micra
37°	185.0 micra
40°	194.9 micra

Blood samples were taken from patients immediately before and immediately after fever treatments lasting three to seven hours at temperatures up to 104°. The following diseases were being treated: schizophrenia, gonorrhea, infectious arthritis, chorea, multiple sclerosis, Parkinson's, asthma and trichinosis. White blood counts before and after five hours of sustained fever at 105° to 106° showed 6,818 and 13,225 respectively with neutrophils being 64 and 80, lymphocytes 20 and 11, monocytes 4 and 3, eosinophils 5 and 2, and basophils 1 and 0.

The "febrile hemogram," pattern of white blood cells after artificial fever, shows an increase in white blood cells after the fever varying with the duration and height of the fever. Notice that increase is not across the board, but selective, indicating the divine principle of economy and efficiency in the body. The peak increase in white blood cells is chiefly from an increase in neutrophils, and may go as high as 40,000.[27] Band forms, immature neutrophils, are not uncommon. When the neutrophil peak has passed, the total white count usually remains high for a few hours first by an increase in monocytes and later by an increase in lymphocytes. Lymphocytes usually show a decrease in number during the actual time of the fever.[28]

Leukocytes, Toxins, and Chemical Attraction

Chemotaxis is a word used for the chemical attraction observed in cells capable of motility. It is a movement either away from or toward a certain chemical, determined by whether the chemical is beneficial or harmful to the cell. This property of cells provides a means of seeking nutrients and more favorable environment; or, as in the case of leukocytes, helps them in the performance of their protective functions. The briskness with which chemotaxis works determines whether a disease-producing germ will be able to invade the tissues of the human host. Bacteria which possess the property of chemotaxis are more successful in invading intestinal tissue than are other bacteria.[29] It has been shown, however, that those germs which ordinarily invade the colon can be attracted to chemotactic substances in the lumen more easily than in the tissue. This property is especially important in the small bowel where contact of the contents with the intestinal wall is brief.[30]

It is likely that proper health of the bowel wall, and proper attention to the techniques of eating food (chewing properly, avoiding overeating, taking small bites, and refraining from drinking with meals) may be of prime importance in preventing any intestinal infection. The secretions of the healthy digestive tract from the mouth to the anus are formidable defenses against bacteria and other microorganisms, killing and digesting them on contact. Yet, even small abuses of the digestive tract weaken its effectiveness and sabotage our defenses. The wise person makes himself knowledgeable about the laws of digestion and faithfully follows them with unwavering discipline, demonstrating his appreciation for this priceless equipment.

The white blood cells are concerned in various defensive and repair functions of the body. They play important roles in protecting the body against invading germs, and in the production of antibodies. Chemotactic properties have been observed chiefly in the neutrophils, but they can be demonstrated also in eosinophils, lymphocytes, and monocytes. It is unfortunate that bacteria also possess chemotaxis, but white blood cells are more powerful and swift and can be relied upon to per-

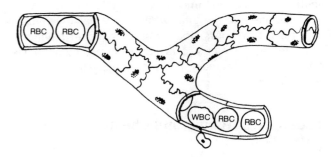

A capillary showing the "shingle" arrangement of its lining cells with "pores" between the cells. Red blood cells are designated RBC and a white blood cell is designated WBC. A normal neutrophil is worming its way through a pore, probably in response to a chemical signal (chemotaxis) from some foreign body or germ outside the capillary. Cortisone, certain other drugs and chemicals, and inherited weaknesses may interfere with the mobility or chemical digestants of white blood cells.

fectly protect us if we do our part. As in the physical, so in the spiritual. While sin is unfortunately with us, "grace doth much more abound." If we flee temptation and surrender to God, we will not be overcome by sin. In the body, white blood cells actually worm their way through blood vessel walls in response to chemotactic substances, giving abundant protection. Chemotaxis is a property of defense in animals and of aggression in bacteria. We can better comprehend many Bible truths by a thorough understanding of our anatomy and physiology.

The influenza virus is reported to be able to reduce the chemotaxis of white blood cells. It is this property that enhances the frequency of bacterial infections after influenza, particularly with staphylococci and pneumococci to produce pneumonia.[31] Fortunately, charcoal can adsorb toxins and some viruses, and hydrotherapy can enhance the motility and responsiveness of leukocytes.

The effect of electricity on natural healing has not been explored as well as the effects of chemical compounds. As long ago as 1860 and 1910 there were research reports of electric currents leaving injured skin. This is called "the current of injury." It is known that certain cells and tissues are electrical conductors and that electrical fields too weak to be picked up on electroencephalogram readings may be common to the brain and may actually regulate the nerve firing, a combination of electrical and chemical events. Anything that disturbs the proper flow of the body's electrical current disturbs the health.

It has been shown that externally applied electrical currents can regenerate amphibian limbs, can assist in the healing of human fractures and ulcers, and even partially regenerate mammalian limbs. In animals who naturally regenerate their limbs, there are large electrical currents that escape from the site of the amputated limb. It is felt that these currents may be the drive behind regeneration, independent of nerves. The sodium concentration seems to be involved. Sodium passing through the membranes of the cells alters large molecules in the membranes, thus promoting wound healing and limb regeneration.[275]

Electric shock can cause a massive outpouring of white blood cells, up to 57,000 within two to four hours.[32] Some think the electric shock may directly stimulate the pituitary-adrenal system in some way. Other factors could be changes in plasma protein concentration, extracellular fluid, and hemoconcentration.

Blood Sedimentation Rate

The sedimentation rate is the speed with which red blood cells in a test tube settle out of liquid blood (clotting having been blocked by anticoagulants). It is controlled by the electrical charge on the membrane which envelops the red blood cells. This charge is partly determined by protein substances suspended in the blood. In disease the blood proteins are altered, the electrical charge is changed, and the *red blood cells stick together* and settle out of the blood more rapidly. In fevers brought on by disease associated with abnormal proteins, there is a rapid rate of sedimentation of red blood cells.

In the fever treatments used in hydrotherapy there are no abnormal proteins produced. "Sedimentation rates were determined on 41 patients who were receiving physically-induced fever. . . . Determinations were made before, during, immediately after, and the day after fever treatments. No significant variations in the sedimentation rates were found in these four determinations. For practical purposes, physically-induced fever used therapeutically does not affect the sedimentation rate."[33] We can assume that reasonable levels of artificial fever do not adversely affect the blood proteins. The blood normally contains a number of protein substances that fight infection, including opsonins, agglutinins, lysins, and complement, along with the antibodies. In disease altering these substances increases the sedimentation rate.

Aspirin Blocks Important Mechanisms

Aspirin inhibits the formation of prostaglandin E in the midbrain. Since prostaglandin E is the agent of the body to set in motion the fever response, giving aspirin blocks a fever. Yet a fever activates several defense mechanisms, and should not be carelessly brought down. If the physiological mechanisms of fighting germs are stimulated at the same time a fever is reduced, the act of bringing down the fever is a result of lessening toxicity, a thing of the body's own doing, and not a blocking pro-

cedure caused by the interference with normal defense mechanisms.[34] [35] [36]

Circadian Rhythms

The body temperature has a diurnal and circadian rhythm as well as a 28 day schedule for both men and women. The thermostat is located in the brain stem. The autonomic nervous system controls the body temperature. Diurnal variations in rectal temperature are about two degrees in normal subjects. The temperature is higher after a meal or exertion, and lower after sleep. Rectal temperature may rise to 103° following strenuous exercise. Conditions that decrease heat production include fasting, sleeping, and short applications of heat that lessen heat production while increasing heat elimination.

The body temperature is one of the factors that we use to recognize health or disease. Although there may be large differences in daily or circadian temperature rhythm from one person to another, the daily responses of a normal individual are consistent. Body temperature peaks at about 6:00 P.M. each day. Six percent of people who regularly take their temperature think they have a fever of unknown origin when in reality they have only slight elevation in body temperature as a normal variant.[27]

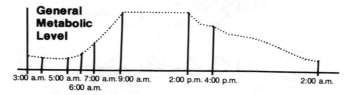

Circadian Rhythm—Normal pattern. At about 3:00 a.m., the hormone and enzyme supports to such functions as muscular strength, cheerfulness, proper thinking patterns, the digestive system, the genito-urinary system, and even respiration, are profoundly reduced. For one who is accustomed to arising at 7:00 a.m. there is a release of ACTH from the pituitary about 5:00 to stimulate the adrenals. By 6:00 adrenalin is being secreted in small quantity to arouse the thyroid, the ovaries or testes, the stomach and pancreas.

Throughout the day there is much benefit to us from these rhythms. Taste, smell, hearing, and reaction to noises and noxious stimuli are all on a circadian rhythm. Pain tolerance is greatly influenced by circadian rhythms as are allergies, physical strength, and sense of well being. Drugs may adversely alter the circadian rhythm, and may reset the time clock, as may also eating off schedule and having a delay in bedtime. Keenness of memory, evenness of disposition, and brightness of intelligence are also enhanced by a proper support from a perfectly programmed circadian rhythm. Protein eaten at 8:00 a.m. rapidly raises the amino acid levels in the blood, but the same meal at 8:00 p.m. does not. By simply inverting the light-dark cycle once a week, one laboratory has shown a significant reduction in the average life span of certain animals.

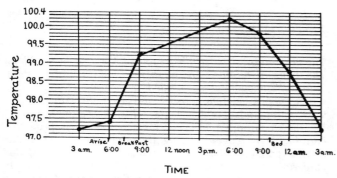

The normal body temperature goes up and down during 24 hours. Exercise, eating, fasting, certain types of hydrotherapy, and ovulation cause the temperature to go up temporarily. Sleeping brings the temperature down.

Normal oral temperature may vary from 96.6° to 100° during the course of 24 hours in the same normal subject. The lowest readings are usually in the morning, between three and five o'clock, when the circadian rhythm is at its lowest ebb. The highest readings are in the late afternoon and evening. For an individual who works at night and sleeps in the daytime, there is a partial reversal of this normal diurnal curve, although the normal swing is not as pronounced, either for the highs or the lows.[38]

Skin temperature may vary normally in the resting person from 90° to 97.6°. If the temperature reading is taken in the axilla, the normal reading is 97.6°. The extremities should not be lower than 90° to 93° except when the person is actively sweating. To allow habitual chilling of the skin causes "cold adaptation" with a series of uncomfortable and unhealthful conditions associated with it. One cannot achieve the optimum level of health if the extremities are habitually chilled. Many women usually carry a skin temperature of the extremities of 80° to 84°, or much lower. At this temperature, potassium and other

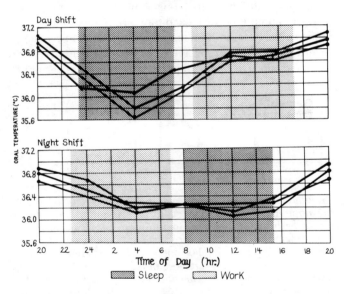

Circadian Rhythm—Night shift worker. Human beings are basically daytime beings in which the general metabolic level is humming most vigorously in the daytime. We are larks, not owls. Those who are more energetic in the evening derive their high spirits from psychological factors, not physiological strength. Costly adjustments must be made to run the equipment at night, and, while these adjustments can be made by the body, it is at the expense of some acceleration of aging.

Night workers are not able to attain a direct reversal of the up and down rhythms of body temperature, hormone production, and other physiologic functions. Instead, night workers tend to flatten out their curves as typified in the contrasting temperature curves above, day shift workers at the top and night shift workers at the bottom.

wastes accumulate in the tissues to be released suddenly on rewarming. Potassium excess in the blood causes heart rhythm disturbances. Many heart rhythm irregularities have their origin in this mechanism, especially those arising after going to bed. The normal temperature of internal organs is about 102° to 104°, although special activity can raise the temperature of these organs to 104° to 107°[25 44]

Anatomy of the Skin: Surface Cells

The marvelous devices of the skin to protect from disease and assist in healing have not been appreciated as they should. Anyone fighting disease who will stimulate, cleanse, warm, and protect the skin will have millions of robust allies in the versatile and talented structures of the skin. The cells on the surface of the skin are flattened, somewhat like shingles, but are laid layer upon layer. At the base of three to ten layers of these cells (stratum germinativum), there is a final sheet of single cells called the stratum basalis. All of this outer portion including the sheet is called the epidermis.

Beneath the epidermis is the dermis. The dermis contains the hair follicles, the sebaceous glands, the erector pili muscles which contract to make "goose flesh,"

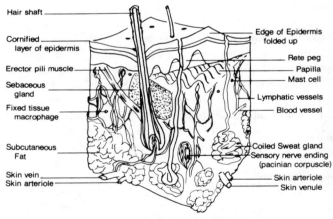

The skin is most wonderfully adapted to perform its function. The hairs in humans are more for touch sensation than warmth. The pacinian corpuscle is a sensory end-organ. The sweat glands excrete wastes and regulate temperature, sebaceous glands produce sebum which keeps the skin pliable, the erector pili muscle contracts to make gooseflesh, the cornified layer prevents drying, the projections on top of the dermis (papillae) fit into depressions on the bottom of the epidermis (rete pegs) to anchor the epidermis and assist with nourishment. Notice the profusion of blood vessels to make a rich area to shunt blood when needed. The subcutaneous fat is for cushioning and storage (excess fat from the blood, toxic metals, alcohol and other substances. Sugar is also temporarily stored in the skin after a meal).

lymphatics, capillaries, nerves and connective tissues. These structures are enormously useful in fighting disease. That they fight quietly should not be misconstrued to mean they are weak or ineffectual.

The muscles of the skin consist of smooth muscle and are involuntary. There is elastic tissue in the skin which holds the skin tight, and helps prevent wrinkling. If all the tiny muscles of the skin contract at one time, as might happen in producing "goose flesh," there is suffi-

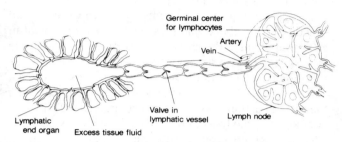

Lymphatic vessel and lymph node. Excess tissue fluid is picked up by the lymphatics, filtered through the lymph node and eventually returned to the blood by a vein in the chest.

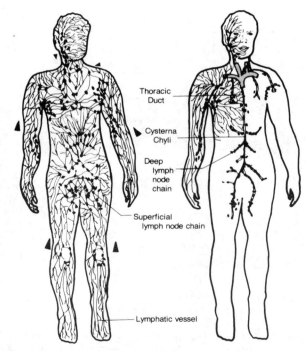

The lymphatic system is a one way system that carries away any excess fluid that may have gotten pushed or pulled out of the capillaries. The direction of flow is shown by the arrows. If it accumulates it is called "edema." Wastes, toxins, and debris are carried out of the tissues with the fluid, necessitating the filtering stations called "lymph nodes." In a smoker the nodes near the lungs become black with carbon dust which comes from the lymphatic fluid in and around the lungs.

cient muscular activity and heat-saving effects to raise the body temperature one or two degrees!

Lymphatics and Edema

The lymphatic vessels are numerous in the dermis. They consist of a one-way system of vessels, carrying away the excess fluid that pushes out of the capillaries with each heart beat. If this fluid is not carried away by the lymphatics, it tends to accumulate. This condition is spoken of as "edema." The lymphatics can carry off large amounts of tissue wastes, toxins, and debris. They can be reflexively activated by the effects of massage on the muscles of the skin itself, as well as on the large muscles of the extremities. Exercise, both active and passive, increases the flow of lymphatic fluid, by massaging the vessels. Their valves direct the fluid on toward the great veins for removal.

Blood Vessels and Nerves

The skin blood vessels are a reservoir capable of holding thirty percent of the total blood volume![39] The skin possesses a specific reacting capacity to antigens *more than ten times* as great as the reaction capacities of the muscles, the brain, or plasma![40] It is this tremendous capacity for altering its physiological responses that gives the skin such an important influence on disease conditions and makes applications to the skin effective in fight-

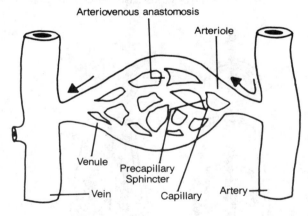

Terminal vascular bed. The intricate capillary networks ramify through all tissues and organs. The precapillary sphincter and the size of the capillary bed (which is greater than the size of the arteriole bed) result normally in a slower blood flow and lower blood pressure in the capillaries than in the arterioles. The arteriovenous anastomoses can open widely and can divert the stream of blood so that it does not continue down the arteriole, but shunts across to the venule and returns to the heart. It is this mechanism that cuts down on blood flow to a part when it becomes chilled, so that the blood will not become dangerously cold.

ing disease. In fever treatment, blood brought from the deep organs to the surface comes in contact with this reacting portion. The Creator designed these healing mechanisms and placed them where we can easily reach them.

All skin applications produce reflexive effects on the blood vessels not only on those directly under the applications, but also on those at some distance. Derivation is the act of drawing blood from a distant, internal part as applications are made over a large area of the surface of the body. As an example, a hot foot bath is a derivative, drawing away blood that may be congesting the head, chest, pelvis, or abdomen. It will not draw blood from non-congested areas as effectively as from congested parts. Retrostasis, the opposite of derivation, is characterized by the production of internal congestion brought on by cold applications over large portions of the body.

The heating compress combines both responses; retrostasis begins immediately and lasts for a few minutes as blood is forced back into blood vessels behind the area of application, then a secondary effect of derivation ensues as the compress heats up. The electrical nerve impulses regulating changes in blood volume in derivation and retrostasis are transmitted through the autonomic nervous system, the nerves and nerve endings to blood vessels, lymph channels, sebaceous and sweat glands, elastic connective tissue, and muscular tissues of the organs and tissues involved. These reactions in skin greatly increase the usefulness of the skin in directing and influencing many activities associated with healing.

Return of Blood to the Heart

Marvelous is the engineering of the human machine. We can see the genius of the Divine Engineer in the method of returning blood to the heart. The muscles of the extremities are very useful in pushing blood along the veins back to the heart. As muscles contract, pressure is put on the blood in the veins, causing the blood to go forward. Backward flow is prevented by the valves in the veins. This is called the muscle pump.

The respiratory movements, and proper tone and function of the abdominal muscles are also beneficial in returning blood to the chest. With each inspiration, there is a negative pressure produced in the chest which results in pulling blood from the abdomen, the neck and head, and the extremities back to the chest. Take note that ". . . the healthy action of the respiratory organs, assisting the circulation of the blood, invigorates the whole system, excites the appetite, promotes digestion, and induces sound, sweet sleep, thus not only refreshing the body, but soothing and tranquilizing the mind."[41]

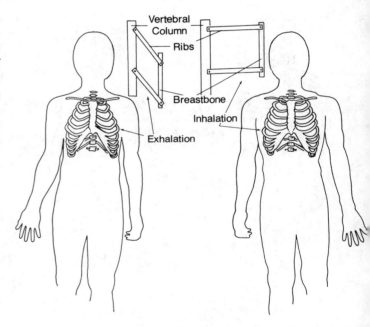

Several factors unite to cause the blood to return to the heart: the hydrostatic pressure from the beat of the heart, tissue pressures from the muscles and other nearby structures, valves in the veins which prevent backflow, and negative pressure in the chest. With each inspiration negative pressure in the chest pulls blood into the chest from the head, gastrointestinal tract, and extremities. The heart counts on this assistance. Full and deep inspirations promote good digestion, clearheadedness, and brisk circulation. With ribs elevated the chest has a much larger capacity than when the ribs are slanted downward, as in the two diagrams of the box.

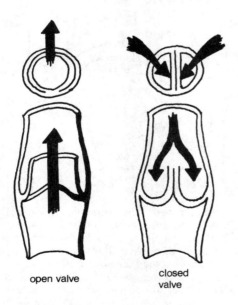

open valve   closed
                              valve

Valves in veins permit only one-way blood flow. In varicose veins the valves are damaged and stretched so they no longer prevent backward flow.

CHAPTER FOUR

Temperature Control

Thermometers

Thermometers for measuring the intensity of heat are divided in scales containing 100 or 180 steps from freezing to boiling of water. The Celsius scale, previously known as centigrade scale, has 100 steps or degrees. The Fahrenheit scale contains 180 degrees. Therefore the Celsius degree is larger, being 9/5 the size of the Fahrenheit degree, and the Fahrenheit degree is 5/9 the size of the Celsius degree. To change Celsius to Fahrenheit one must first multiply by 9/5. This gives the number of Fahrenheit degrees above the freezing point. Since the Fahrenheit scale begins at 32, this number should be added to the result to obtain the correct Fahrenheit reading. To change Fahrenheit to Celsius, subtract 32, and multiply the remainder by 5/9.

Conversion Table
TEMPERATURE

°F	°C	°C	°F
0	-17.8	0	32.0
95	35.0	35.	95.0
96	35.6	35.5	95.9
97	36.1	36.	96.8
98	36.7	36.5	97.7
99	37.2	37.	98.6
100	37.8	37.5	99.5
101	38.3	38.	100.4
102	38.9	38.5	101.3
103	39.4	39.	102.2
104	40.0	39.5	103.1
105	40.6	40.	104.0
106	41.1	40.5	104.9
107	41.7	41.	105.8
108	42.2	41.5	106.7
109	42.8	42.	107.6
110	43.3	100	212

°F to °C: 5/9 (°F − 32)   °C to °F: (9/5 × °C) + 32

Temperature references in this book will be in Fahrenheit readings unless specifically noted otherwise. To change 40° Celsius to Fahrenheit, multiply by 9 and divide by 5, then add 32, resulting in 104° F. To change 104° Fahrenheit to Celsius, first subtract 32, which gives 72, multiply by 5, and divide by 9 to obtain Celsius reading of 40.

There are several good places in the body to determine temperature. The usual sites and readings for taking body temperature are: oral (98.6°), axillary or underarm (97.6°), and rectal (99.6°). The subject should not have hot or cold food or liquid in the mouth for at least ten minutes before measuring oral temperature. Mouth breathing and talking also affect oral temperature readings. The thermometer should be left in the mouth, under the tongue, with the mouth closed and the subject not talking, for three to five minutes to obtain the most accurate reading. If one obtains a reading after one minute and allows the thermometer to stay in place for one additional minute and detects no change in reading, an accurate temperature reading probably has been achieved.

Sweating and Temperature Regulation

Approximately 11,000 square feet are represented by the combined surface of the ducts of the sweat glands! Such a large area for excreting materials should not be overlooked in the application of natural remedies. It is a fact that poor habits and environmental situations can cause unresponsive, unhealthy sweat glands. The secretion of the sweat glands is about 98% water and 2% solids. By contrast, the urine is only 96% water but 4% solids, both organic and inorganic wastes, illustrating how much impurities the skin can carry off. About one pint of fluid and impurities are lost in each eight hour period by a person when not obviously sweating. In certain diseases, there are some toxic waste products that are more readily handled by the skin than by the kidneys.

The total amount of water excreted by the skin in any given length of time is approximately twice that given off by the lungs. During heating treatments, in order to encourage the patient to sweat profusely, hot drinks and copious quantities of water should be given before and during the treatment. Some individuals even require hot drinks in order to secure free perspiration.

The rate of obvious sweating in cold weather is essentially zero. When a person first begins to be exposed to hot weather, he can sweat only about 1.5 liters per hour; within ten days he can double that amount. In six weeks he has increased his sweating ability to $2\frac{1}{2}$ times the rate of his unconditioned state. During maximal sweating a person could lose up to 8 pounds of weight per hour. When the rate of sweating is low, most of the sodium chloride (NaCl) is reabsorbed from the secretion so that little or none is lost. When sweat production is heavy in the unacclimatized person, the rate of NaCl reabsorption does not increase accordingly, so that the sweat may contain more NaCl, and can rise almost to the level in the sweat that it is in the plasma. Other substances lost in sweat are urea, lactic acid, and potassium. More urea is lost when the sweat rate is high than when it is low. Aldosterone (from adrenals and gonads) causes less sodium to be lost in the sweat. It is beneficial to have at least one sweating experience per day to get rid of wastes and mineral buildup. Wastes can be reabsorbed into the blood from the clothing and skin if they are not washed regularly, placing an extra burden on the body to re-excrete them.

A large number of sweat glands may become permanently inactivated during childhood if they are never vigorously stimulated by heating or exercise. It is apparently injurious to sweat glands for a child to be reared in air-conditioning. If, however, the child lives in the tropics, or exercises briskly in the out-of-doors, all the sweat glands present at birth become activated during childhood and youth and remain so throughout life.

It will be remembered that Adam and Eve were given coats to replace the aprons they had hastily fashioned. The skin apparently performs its functions better if it is kept covered, even in Edenic subtropical climates. Although the mechanism is poorly understood, sixty percent of the loss of heat of a lightly clothed body occurs by radiation of infrared rays from the surface of the body. Since the body ceases to emit infrared rays when one is in direct sunshine, clothing the body helps to keep the body cool by limiting its exposure to the infrared rays from the sun and encouraging heat loss by radiation of infrared.

At ordinary room temperatures, evaporation ac-

counts for about 25% of heat loss from the body. When the environmental temperature is higher, evaporation is one of the main ways the body loses heat. Humidity decreases the rate of evaporation. In summer the proper type of clothing increases the rate of evaporation, especially if air currents are capable of moving freely around a person.

Perspiration during a heating treatment may be two to three pints per hour. Perspiration is increased by an increase in body temperature, an increase in the heart action, drinking much water, the use of percussion and friction with the treatment, the use of certain drugs and nervous stimulation. Perspiration may be decreased by cold, by reduced water intake, drugs taken, such diseases as

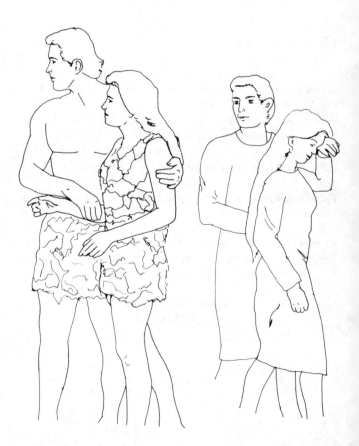

The wisdom of the Creator is illustrated by the provision of coats of skins to replace the aprons of fig leaves they made for themselves after losing the protective robe of light they possessed before their sin. Protection from the now unfriendly climate and animals, and accidents due to reduced sensitivity of the senses was necessary. Even in an ideal climate both men and women probably find comfort and healthfulness promoted by extensive protection of the skin with clothing, both summer and winter. In winter, clothing should be designed so that heat accumulates, in summer so that heat dissipates.

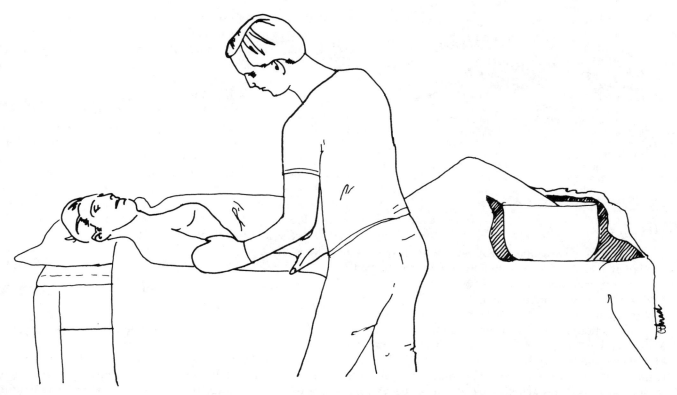

Preparing for a cold mitten friction by giving a hot foot bath. All cold applications should be administered only to warm persons. With your own hand actually check the temperature of the extremities before giving a cold treatment. If the skin is not warm, first use a heating treatment such as a hot foot bath.

cancer or paralysis, and by increased kidney or bowel output (which is often reciprocal with the skin).

Prolonged or frequently repeated sweating, artificially induced, weakens the skin and reduces its power to withstand cold, unless it is counteracted by the frequent application of cold compresses. An important point for the hydrotherapist to remember is that the skin should be prepared for a cold application by an increase in skin temperature.

Heat Conservation and Dissipation

The heat conservation processes in the body include shivering, contraction of the erector pili muscles, and contraction of surface blood vessels causing the blood to go from the skin to the deeper tissues. During a fever the skin surface temperatures, particularly the temperature of the toes, may remain the same as before the fever, or may get even cooler, while the internal temperature is being elevated. This phenomenon is due to constriction of blood vessels in the skin and dilatation of blood vessels deep within the body in heat conservation. After the elevation of internal temperature, the skin surface temperature gradually rises.[43] Assumption of heat conservation posture may involve folding the arms or holding them close to the body, closing the hands, squatting or curling the body into a ball with the legs up against the thighs, and shallow breathing. In heat conservation the skin is usually dry.

When the body shifts from heat conservation to heat dissipation (the fever is about to go down), there is a reversal of the above-mentioned features. The skin blood vessels open up and begin to carry much blood and the skin becomes flushed. The sweat glands produce copiously, and the skin becomes moist. The body posture straightens out and the palms, trunk and thighs are uncurled and the arms held away from the body or over the head. Respiration becomes deep, with loss of much heat with each exhalation.

In a fever, in addition to a chill, goose flesh, typical posture, and shallow breathing, there may be excessive thirst, malaise, backache, insomnia, headache, delirium and other nervous symptoms. There is often increased pulse rate and cardiac output, chill or chilliness, loss of appetite, foul breath, coated tongue, hot and dry skin, or cold and clammy skin, constipation or diarrhea, and scanty, highly-colored urine.

**Normal Body Temperatures:
Surface and Internal**[44]

Tip of ear 83.64°	Cheek 93.92°
Breast 88°	Pectoral region, over
Back of hand 90.5	muscle, 94.5°
to 91.76°	Hollow of closed hand
Calf 92.5°	94.64 to 96.18°
Forehead 93.38 to 93.92°	Rectum 100°
Upper part of thigh 93.6°	Blood, average 102°
Forearm 93.7°	Brain 104°
Sternum 93.9°	Right ventricle 106°
Right iliac fossa 93.9°	Liver 106.5°
Hollow of open hand	Left ventricle 107°
93.9 to 94.6°	

Heat Stroke

If not caught early and wisely dealt with, heat stroke can be fatal. Heat stroke is a condition in which the body temperature continues to rise out of control even up to 112° at which point protein breakdown occurs, followed rapidly by death. Body heat accumulates when the total heat production exceeds heat dissipation. If the situation is progressive, heat stroke will result. It is caused by a high work rate in very hot and humid conditions. If the ability of the body to lose heat is compromised for any reason, such as drugs or pulmonary disease, heat stroke develops in less extreme conditions. Dehydration predisposes to heat stroke by decreasing the efficiency of evaporation of sweat which results in reduction of cooling of the skin surface.[45] Also, the circulation is not as brisk if there is dehydration.

Circumstances that can increase the likelihood of heat stroke are obesity, cardiovascular disease, being unaccustomed to heat and humidity, advanced age, and alcoholism. The absence of sweating is regarded as an essential feature in the diagnosis of heat stroke. Heat stroke mortality is about 80% or more. Heat exhaustion acts somewhat like heat stroke, but sweating is always present.

Other conditions which can cause a sustained fever are malignancies, intracranial tumors, increased thyroid activity, heat exhaustion (in response to heat or in response to anesthesia), and the adrenal tumor, pheochromocytoma.[46] Damage to the body tissues in ordinary fevers is due to the toxic effects of the germs or other fever-producing agents, not from the increased temperature itself, until after the temperature reaches 108° by mouth. Artificial fevers have been taken that high in some experimental medical centers without serious tissue injury. A natural fever is usually a sign of an injurious agent; it is not itself the injurious agent.

The limits of tolerance of body temperature have a range on both the low and high sides from about 77° to 111°. At 110° to 111°, the individual loses consciousness.

At 112° there are irreversible protein denaturations that occur in most body cells. There is also a typical response of the body and mind while the temperature is falling below normal. As the temperature falls, the person loses consciousness at about 92°. There is often cardiac fibrillation at 82°, with death invariably at 77°.[47]

Conditions that decrease heat production include fasting, sleeping, and short applications of heat that lessen heat production while increasing heat elimination. Subnormal temperatures may be obtained also in cases of hemorrhage, shock, dehydration, poor oxygen supply, low thyroid activity, exhaustion, exposure while inadequately clothed, and small neck and jaw structure which allows the blood from the carotid arteries to cool as it travels to the mouth where the temperature will be measured.

Adaptive, Pyrogenic, and Artificial Fevers

There are three types of fevers: (1) adaptive—from work, climate, hormones, etc., (2) pyrogenic—from disease, and (3) artificial—caused by application of external heat to deliberately elevate the temperature. As generally used, the term fever refers to an elevation of temperature caused by any kind of agent. The moderately elevated body temperature is not itself injurious, but the agent may be. Pyrogens, the substances that cause fevers, circulate and influence the thermostat in the brain.

Germs are not the sole causes of fever. Any damaged tissue, whether from operations, injuries, foreign proteins, or toxic chemicals, can act as pyrogens to cause an increase in body heat. There are certain lesions of the brain which interfere with the thermostatic mechanism, and cause an elevation in body temperature. Cancer and leukemia, because of an increase in basal metabolic rate, as well as the presence of pyrogenic substances that can result from tissue destruction, can cause an elevation of body heat.

A small amount of milk seepage into the blood stream can cause a lactating woman to have a high fever. A very small number of typhoid bacilli in the blood stream can cause a raging fever. Any foreign protein in the blood stream can act as a pyrogen and may quickly elevate the body temperature.

Pyrogens affect the thermoregulatory mechanism in an unknown way to cause the body to change gears and begin to conserve heat. Pyrogens are the actual toxins themselves, or the products of tissue injury, the split protein products from the injured cells being absorbed into the blood. As the blood circulates, the altered protein products stimulate the thermostat in the hypothalamus to set in the motion the heat conservation mechanisms of the body. Split products of protein breakdown are produced in infections, malignancy, injury and stress.

Causes of Fevers

1. Infection (many bacteria, some viruses, Rickettsias, protozoa, fungi).

2. Cancer, especially lymphomas, notably Hodgkin's disease.

3. Tissue death (chemical or mechanical injuries, myocardial infarction, pulmonary embolism).

4. Foreign proteins in the blood (lactation, venomous bites, intestinal absorption).

5. Dehydration (water deprivation, excessive sweating, heat treatments)

6. Increased thyroid activity

7. Muscular or chemical activity

Fever Is a Friend

Fever is a symptom and is not an enemy, but a friend. In many infections, fever enhances the defense mechanisms. It is certain that in various types of syphilis, fever has a profoundly beneficial effect. In viral infections, interferon production is either reduced or increased as the temperature goes up or down. It is recognized that the outcome of polio virus infection is favorably influenced by a higher body temperature. Therefore, the use of drugs in infections to bring the fever down has unexpected disadvantages.

In 1957 Isaacs and Lindenmann were studying the resistance that a person has to a second virus when one already has one viral disease. They discovered a group of substances which they named interferons. These are substances of low molecular weight, glycoproteins, and are produced at the onset of an infection by a virus. They actually *precede antibody formation* against the virus. Therefore, while the body is cranking up its antibody-forming cells the interferons are already being produced. These glycoproteins are not specific for one virus, but the interferons produced by a certain illness act as agents *against all viruses,* in contrast to antibodies that act only against the very virus that the antibody is made to match, and only that one.

Interferons inhibit cancer producing viruses, have interactions with the immune systems, induce enzymes to be produced inside of cells, and have a direct inhibition on tumor cell growth. They have been used in the treatment of herpes simplex, varicella, herpes zoster, juvenile laryngeal papillomas, condyloma acuminatum, influenza A, hepatitis B, rabies and chronic active hepatitis. They have been used against such malignancies as melanoma, multiple myeloma, osteogenic sarcoma, and cervical and breast cancer.

Three types of human interferons have been distinguished: (1) those that are prepared by white blood cells, (2) those that are made by fibroblasts and (3) those that are prepared from lymphoblastoid cells. All of these are known as Type I interferons and are primarily antiviral in their action. There is a Type II interferon which involves the cells of the immune system. Species specificity is another property of interferons, that is, a human produces human cell interferon and the use of animal interferon will cause reactions in humans just as using animal blood will cause a transfusion reaction in humans.[48]

Success in treating disease is usually due to attention to many small matters. These matters are not mysterious, but do require energy, attention and carefulness. In treating fevers it is well to remember that the body temperature is increased by dehydration, prolonged heavy exercise, labor of childbirth, work in hot environments, various drugs and chemicals, pyrogens, toxins, cancers, hyperthyroidism, stress, fear, excitement and so forth. "Drug fever" can occur from taking any kind of medication.

The temperature of a small infant may fall by as much as seven degrees during a cold bath. A crying spell may cause the temperature to rise by two or three degrees. We had an infant whose mother reported that she could not get a simple teething fever down by the baths we had prescribed. On investigation it was found that the baby was dehydrated. Correcting that simple matter made a much happier baby whose fever promptly responded to the usual methods.

Public speakers notice that they become dehydrated after several hours of speaking, and that the body temperature is slightly elevated. The cause for both the dehydration and the temperature elevation is anxiety, sometimes called "psychogenic fever." The action of adrenalin may be at the root of this kind of fever.

During fevers, because of certain complicated body reactions having to do with respiration and the formation of urine, chlorides may be retained in the body which causes a retention of water. Because of this water retention, the *body weight may actually increase during a fever.* As soon as the fever goes down, the chlorides are lost, and there is a diuresis, resulting in a sudden drop in weight.[50]

It was discovered that very hot baths cause a 10% fall in blood cholesterol, a 10% rise in blood sugar, but have no effect on urea. With hot baths there is a slight rise in systolic blood pressure and a great drop in diastolic blood pressure, both of temporary duration.[51] It should be borne in mind that the heart rate is increased by many of the same factors that increase body temperature including the following: dehydration, blood loss, prolonged heavy exercise, anemia, obstetrical labor and delivery, work in hot temperatures, pyrogens, stress, fear, excitement and hyperthyroidism.

When cool showers are used after routine whirlpool therapy or exercises in a warm water pool there is a statistically significant increase in the diastolic blood pressure following the cooling shower. There is a significant drop in the mean blood pressure on entering the warm water, followed by a rise in blood pressure associated with the cooling shower. In 5% of patients, the mean blood pressure falls or rises more than 15 millimeters.[52]

Artificial fever produced by baths or other external applications of heat has several effects useful in fighting disease.

Useful Effects of Artificial Fever

1. The white blood cells increase in the peripheral blood.

2. Chemical substances that cause foreign elements and bacteria to be more easily phagocytized by macrophages or leukocytes are released from white blood cells.

3. Blood flushes the skin where fixed macrophages can help purify the blood and add chemicals that make germs easier to destroy.

4. Removal of wastes from the blood is facilitated in the skin.

5. Heat conserving mechanisms are reversed and heat dissipating mechanisms are activated:
    A. Flushing of the skin

    B. Opening of hands, abduction of limbs

    C. Sweating

    D. Deep breathing

    E. Relaxation of muscle tension, shivering, and goose flesh.

Fever and Home Remedies

Recent evidence suggests that with infection fever may enhance survival in an animal model.[53] It was demonstrated that certain lizards survived bacterial infections better if they crawled into the sun and raised the body temperature to 41 or 42° C. At these temperatures, less than 33% die. However, if the lizards are prevented ar-

tificially (by aspirin) from achieving the rise in temperature, 75% or more die of the infection.[54]

The level of fever is determined by the severity of the pathologic process and the strength of the host's reaction. Children and old people may respond with either a greater or lesser temperature reading than healthy adults.

The pulse increases about ten beats per minute for each degree elevation in temperature; exceptions are noted in conditions associated with an increase in intracranial pressure, meningitis, and in typhoid fever, in which cases the pulse is lower than expected for the degree of fever. This reaction of the pulse is an important diagnostic sign in these three disorders, and should not be overlooked. There is an increase in basal metabolic rate of about 7% for each degree elevation of temperature. The toxicity associated with fever may cause restlessness, somnolence, delirium, stupor and coma.

Sweating begins when a downward trend in the temperature occurs. "Lysis" indicates the gradual drop in fever as in recovery from typhoid or childbirth. "Crisis" refers to the abrupt drop in fever as with clearing lobar pneumonia.

Fever is of four types: *continuous:* that fever which is elevated all during the day; *intermittent:* daily fluctuations of two degrees or more as in tuberculosis, Hodgkin's, or coccal septicemia; *remittent:* normal, then up again as in tertian malaria; and *recurring* (relapsing): several days of normal temperature followed by several

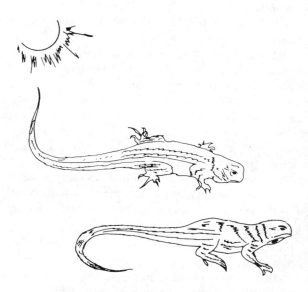

When lizards get an infection they crawl into the sunshine to elevate the body temperature. If the temperature elevation is blocked by aspirin, more than 75% die, illustrating the beneficial function of fever in the defense effort of the body.

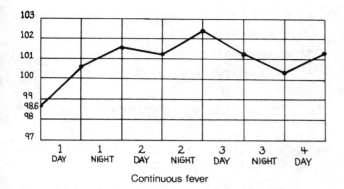

Continuous fever

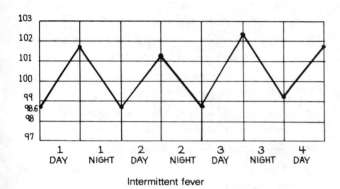

Intermittent fever

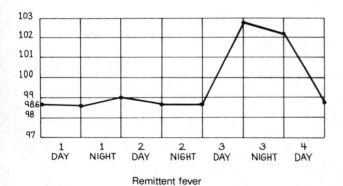

Remittent fever

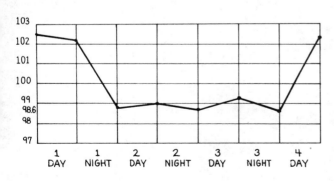

Recurring (Relapsing) fever

days of elevated temperature as in "relapsing fever," Brucellosis, and sometimes Hodgkin's.

The best treatment of fever is alternating hot and cold applications, hot half baths, tepid baths, or infrequently, applications of cool or cold compresses. The first two are preferred, as they also treat the underlying infection by activating white blood cells and immune systems, not just "treating the fever" as drugs do. In natural fevers there is a dilatation of internal blood vessels and constriction of skin blood vessels. The application of cold to the skin increases these conditions, whereas heat reverses them, helps with the oxidation of toxins, and increases blood flow to the surface vessels of the skin where macrophages are permanently stationed. Heating the surface of the skin increases the ability of the phagocytes to destroy the germs, and to detoxify the blood. Probably these cells secrete a specific substance which acts as a strong stimulus to the immune system, increasing antibodies so that larger quantities of bacterial poisons can be eliminated.

Any cold application prolonged over 15 or 20 minutes can cause marked internal congestion. The forcible reduction of temperature in fevers by ice water applications is usually not wise. In congestive heart failure it is especially important not to induce internal congestion. In these patients check the backs of the arms and feet for proper warmth of the body, as chilled skin can cause much blood to transfer to the heart and internal organs, placing an extra burden on these organs.

When giving an enema, either hot or cold, retrostasis or backward congestion, which is expected from the treatment, may cause an increase in blood volume in the chest and abdomen, a vascular compartment already overloaded in the severely handicapped cardiac. Use neutral temperature for enemas in these cases. Note another precaution in using ice cold treatments: avoid extreme cold to the chest in cardiac asthma. An acute attack of cardiac asthma can be precipitated by cold applications to the chest with the resultant retrostasis of blood into the chest.

For children, a full immersion bath is very efficient in the treatment of a fever. For an adult a full immersion bath is simulated by sitting in the full bathtub with wet towels spread over the knees and across the shoulders and chest. The towels may be kept constantly wet by the water from the tub.

Even if the temperature is elevated to 104°, a brief exposure to a hot water bath or fomentations will often treat the underlying infection, bring the blood to the surface, relax the muscles, increase the depth of respiration, and reduce the fever.

Physical cooling methods to reduce fever may be exhausting to the patient—by shivering and other physiologic responses—reducing the strength of the patient to fight the basic disease. In severe illnesses like typhoid fever, an actual harmful effect may result from cold applied to the patient.[49]

Using Water to Reduce Fever

If the *fever is 106° or above,* follow this procedure:

1. A tepid or cool bath, or the hot evaporating sheet pack, with or without rubbing the skin.
2. Cold compress to head and neck.
3. Ice bag or cold compress to the heart in a feeble patient.
4. Cool (95°) rectal irrigation or enema.
5. Fresh, cool (60° to 65°) air in the sickroom.
6. Cool water (60° or tap temperature) taken by mouth to promote sweating.

If the *fever is 103° to 105°* use *one* of the following procedures instead of #1 above; then proceed with #2 to #6 above:

1. Hot blanket pack of short duration (5 to 10 minutes) to reduce the sensation of chilliness and initiate heat dissipating mechanisms.

2. Short hot bath or repeated hot sponging to bring blood to the surface.
3. Hot evaporating sheet pack.
4. Hot fomentations to the abdomen or spine for five to seven minutes.
5. Cold mitten friction or hot mitten friction.

If the *fever is mild, 99° to 103°,* produce an artificial fever by *one* of the following methods:

1. Hot half bath, prolonged to the point of elevating the oral temperature to 102° to 104°. Finish the bath with a pail pour of cold water and a dry friction rub, or cold mitten friction.
2. Russian or electric light bath to the same degree of fever and with the same finish.
3. Hot foot bath with blanket pack, to elevate temperature. Finish off as above.
4. Hot fomentations to chest and spine with cold mitten friction at the end.
5. Hot water or tea to promote sweating.
6. Measures #2 to #6 listed above under treatment of a fever of 106°.

CHAPTER FIVE

CIRCULATORY, NEUROLOGIC AND METABOLIC FACTORS IN HEALING

Lymph Flow

Completely independently of the closed circuit of vessels for the circulation of the blood, there is a one-way system of vessels for the drainage of lymph fluid from the tissues of the body. The lymph fluid is actually blood plasma which accumulates in the tissues as blood circulates and "leaks" its fluid out of the capillaries to bathe the cells near the blood vessels. The excess fluid is expressed from the higher pressure tissues into the very low pressure lymph vessels by the pressure of the tissue itself, by hydrostatic pressure, and by the movement of muscles. Both active and passive motion, such as in massage, can increase the flow of lymph. This emphasizes the necessity of giving passive exercise by means of massage or manipulation when the patient is unable to exercise for himself. About one-thirteenth of the body weight is blood and one-fourth to one-third of that is lymph. Almost this entire quantity of fluid is influenced when hydrotherapy is used. Because of the circulation of blood and lymph, the result of the treatment can be felt all over the body, not just in the part treated.

Reaction Types

Since the body goes through several steps in its reaction to heat or cold, we can speak of the phases in separate groups. There are three phases of reaction: circulatory, nervous and metabolic. In the circulatory reaction the skin becomes reddened because of an increase in blood flow to the skin. Because of the increase in neuromuscular transmission we speak of a nervous system reaction. Metabolic changes in the tissues resulting from the reactions to heat or cold, and the efforts to produce more or less heat dominate certain aspects and constitute the metabolic reaction to temperature change. The circulato-

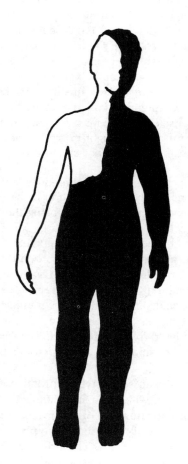

The lymphatic drainage system of the body is part of the defense mechanism. The light area is drained by a system that serves only the right side from the waist up, collecting into the right lymphatic duct. All the rest of the body drains into the thoracic duct as indicated by the black area representing the rest of the body. The lymphatics carry not only fluid but also germs, foreign particles, fat from the digestive tract, fungi, and other substances.

ry phase is usually most pronounced and obvious. It is the phase with which hydrotherapists are most immediately concerned. If the treatment fails to produce a vigorous surface circulation it is said to be an "incomplete reaction." As a treatment continues, a certain degree of fatigue or slowing of the reactive powers develops. At this point, in order to maintain the same degree of reaction possible to obtain at the first of the treatment, the latter applications must be more intense, accompanied by friction, or more prolonged. Percussion may also be used to intensify the reaction.

In order that the reactions not be hindered, the hydrotherapist must give attention to the temperature of the air of the sickroom, the patient, as well as to the water used. One should not trust to his own sensation. The room temperature in winter should be adjusted with a room thermometer to about 65° (60° in fevers is not too low, and some elderly and feeble patients will require higher temperatures). The sick room is generally kept too warm and increases the depression of the patient. In the heat of summer, a room can be kept cool by proper attention to shading from direct sunshine, by hanging wet sheets in the room and circulating air past them, and by the judicious use of electric fans. Air conditioners should be used *only* if air is brought in fresh from the outside continuously, and they do not create a draft on the patient.

Metabolic action can be altered by hydrotherapy, cold producing increased elimination of carbon dioxide (CO_2) and heat; after initially increasing the elimination of CO_2, the cold eventually reduces it. Alkalinity of the blood favors the action of white blood cells in eating germs, while acidosis inhibits it. Carbonic acid is produced in the transfer of CO_2 from tissues to the lungs. The overbreathing which accompanies hydrotherapy reduces this acid, and through a complicated process results in alkalizing the blood, bringing the conditions most favorable to phagocytosis.[55] Either excitation or sedation can be obtained by using some form of hydrotherapy.

A stimulus is an action which produces a response. The application of water as a stimulant is determined by its temperature, the duration of application, and the force or method by which it is applied. The physical response may be positive or negative. The primary effect may be decidedly stimulating and the secondary effect may be quite sedating, even depressing. If an exciting effect on the circulation of the blood and a tonic effect on the heart and blood vessels is desired, water should be used considerably above or below the temperature of the body surface. On the other hand, a neutral bath from 94° to 96° in which one could stay for hours, produces a sedating effect. The duration of the neutral bath may be from one

to even several hours a day. The most disturbed or uncooperative patient, as a rule, soon comes to enjoy its comfort, a real advance in the treatment of mentally ill patients.

During a bath the skin takes up only about 50 to 100 grams of water (up to one-half cupful) during the first 30 minutes, and thereafter does not take up water. The blood pH may be somewhat affected during a bath by the metabolic changes in tissue and by altered breathing of the patient. Marked overbreathing is noted at first; it is more intense the hotter the bath, amounting sometimes to air hunger. This overbreathing can reduce acidosis in diabetes but in normal metabolic states, if prolonged, it can produce the hyperventilation syndrome, with tightening of the muscles, cramps, and emotional distress.

Before the turn of the century, a prominent health journal carried the following statement: "Invalids have frequently used water [treatments] injudiciously, especially if they are extremists. They may not have a correct knowledge of the use of water."[56] The suggested method for the judicious use of water was outlined: (1) Use water not too hot or too cold, (2) always "reduce" the hot bath with cold applications, (3) avoid chilling immediately after the bath; allow no exposure to cold drafts or cold air, and (4) lie down for the reaction for 30 to 60 minutes, or engage in vigorous work or a walk to improve the reaction and prevent chilliness.

Infections and Inflammations

"Infection" is a term that refers to the invasion of the body by an infecting organism or germ such as a virus, bacterium, fungus, or parasite (the latter is spoken of as an infestation). An *"inflammation"* is a response on the part of the body to any kind of injury including infections, and presents with four cardinal signs: rubor, calor, dolor, and tumor (redness, heat, pain and swelling).

In fighting an injury or in clearing up debris, the body first opens up blood vessels in the area through mechanisms located at the site of the injury and is promptly assisted by blood vessel forces acting through the central nervous system. Then the body begins to produce specific weapons to combat the injury, such as antibodies to counteract the chemicals of infection; histamine to counteract the effect of mechanical injury, toxin or hemorrhage; enzymes to counteract or dissolve toxic proteins or foreign objects, etc. While these reactions are occurring, large numbers of white blood cells are called into the area through chemotaxis, or chemical attraction.

Within a few hours, literally millions of white blood cells have moved into the area. The increase in chemical content, blood flow, and white blood cell migration result in swelling, the evidence that the body has moved its big artillery into the area of inflammation.

While the body can usually handle things by itself, it will be greatly assisted by the use of some simple measures from the outside: the application of heat and cold, massages, poultices to reduce the swelling or carry off toxins, plenty of water inside and outside for cleansing and ease in transportation of cells and supplies, just the proper quantity and quality of nutrients to make repairs and provide raw materials, an astringent for microscopic cracks or sutures for large cuts to pull wound edges together, and other assists from without.

A "derivative" may be used to temporarily relieve circulatory congestion by pulling blood from the area of inflammation for cleansing and renewal of the blood, and for refreshing and relief of the patient. The derivative is of great help in any inflammatory or infectious process where swelling or congestion of blood vessels is a feature. It serves to renew the troops on the front lines, bring in fresh supplies, and reduce discomfort.

Not all inflammations are due to bacteria; the mastitis of nursing is rarely due to bacteria, but generally to the escape of small quantities of milk from the ducts into the tissues. Inflammation may be acute or chronic. The term "acute" means that it is of recent origin, continuing to develop, and has not reached a stable point. "Chronic" implies an older affliction; one that may have been worse and has settled down to a stable, unhealed condition; or an inflammatory lesion that is not being successfully dealt with by the body.

CHAPTER SIX

The Prompt and Beneficial Effects of Cold

Cold Causes Paleness and Reddening

The *primary action* of cold causes contraction of blood vessels and reduced blood flow with resultant paleness. The *reaction* to cold brings opening of the blood vessels, increased amounts of blood in the capillaries, and flushing. Percussion and friction both have the same *action* and *reaction* as cold. With the initial striking or forceful stroking comes contraction of blood vessels, but with continuation of the mechanical stimulation there is dilatation of blood vessels and reddening.

If both cold and friction are used together the effect is more pleasant and beneficial than if either is used alone. A plunge into a forceful cold shower while vigorously rubbing the skin is less uncomfortable than easing gradually into a fine, soft spray, as the mechanical effect tends to cause the nerves to become more quickly tolerant of the cold. Rubbing the skin at the point of contact with the shower hastens the adaptation. Cold given as a short (1-4 seconds) and intense (40° to 60°) treatment causes blood vessel *contraction,* but prolonged (5 minutes) and moderate (65° to 80°) causes *dilatation* of blood vessels.

Amount and Rate of Blood Flow at Falling Temperatures

As skin temperature falls, there is a fall in total skin blood flow to the level of 16° C., meaning that the blood vessels progressively contract until the skin temperature reaches 16° C. At that point the total blood flow increases, while capillary flow rate is still very low. The additional blood flow apparently occurs through arteriovenous anastomoses.[57] It is this mechanism that makes cold skin first get red from the increased size of

the vessels, then bluish from the slow rate of blood flow through the capillaries.

Information that the body is cold is received through the central nervous system sensing apparatus as a threat to the body's safety. If the body becomes thoroughly chilled, its various functions are seriously slowed or depressed. Respirations and pulse are less rapid. Toxic waste products accumulate in the tissues. The circulation is profoundly affected. It is therefore readily understood that the body must maintain its temperature at an ideal level in order to properly carry on its various functions. Digestion is a prime example of this effect, since chemical reactions all proceed at a slower rate as the temperature falls.

Injury from Cold

If the body does not get actually chilled, but only receives the sensation of coldness, it will react as if to cold; yet no depression of function or tissue injury occur since there has been no actual chilling of the body fluids to cause a reduction in such processes as digestion, circulation, respiration, and various other functions.

Therefore in hydrotherapy, we may use the sensation of chilliness to bring about a physiologic stimulation, while not allowing the injurious effects of chilling. Such a sensation causes the body to react as if fighting cold by increasing its protective and metabolic activities. Sedentary and elderly persons can be especially benefited by daily cold baths. They can thereby fortify themselves against colds and other infections.

Dr. Hans Selye has used chilling as one of the stress factors in animal experimentation to document and illustrate his theories about the *general adaptation syndrome* and the effects of stress on the body reactions.[54]

31

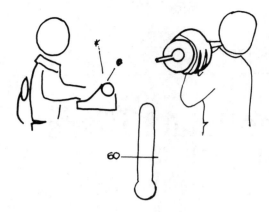

When the thermometer reads 60-below, plan your work according and get the heavy work done. Physical dexterity is decreased with chilling of the muscles, but strength of the muscles is increased.

Cold treatments are contraindicated in the patient who manifests an undue fear of the application, or in a patient who is chilled to any degree. If the patient begins to feel chilled, cold applications should be stopped, or a hot foot bath or hot pack to the spine should be used along with the cold treatment.

Useful Reactions to Cold

Cold applied to the chest over the heart for prolonged periods causes the heart rate to diminish, although rarely below 50 beats per minute. Cold applications of short duration to the same area cause the heart rate to increase.

Dexterity decreases as the skin temperature of the hand falls to 50°. When the temperature of a muscle is reduced to 21° C. (69.8°) the latent time of muscle contraction is elongated and contraction time and relaxation time are both prolonged, reducing the rapidity with which movements can be made.

While dexterity is decreased, strength of muscles is greatly increased by cold.[60] Seventeen subjects were given leg baths which extended to mid-thigh at a mean temperature of 54° for 30 minutes. Each subject was tested for leg strength eleven times during each session. The eleven measurements were taken immediately before and after the treatment, and every 20 minutes for three hours after the treatment, while the subject was relaxing in the laboratory. The effect observed was that of increasing isometric strength by prolonged cold. Both vasodilatation and increased blood flow occurred. The effects lasted as long as six hours. Cold delayed the onset of fatigue.

It was felt that the increased strength was due to in-

creased blood flow to the deep muscles caused by restriction of peripheral blood flow during the treatment. Cold suppresses the inhibitory factors that set the upper limits of maximal voluntary contractions of human muscle. The conclusion of the experiment was that the 30 minute cold bath increases the voluntary maximal lifting strength of the legs. This effect can be used to good advantage in disorders characterized by muscle weakness, such as poliomyelitis, atrophy, multiple sclerosis, muscular dystrophy, strokes, and paralysis.

Exposure to cold is able to reinforce the action of the extensor groups (wrists and fingers, ankles, etc.). In treating a weak or paralyzed hand or foot it should be immersed from three to six times, approximately 3 seconds each time in water maintained at a temperature between 35° and 40° by the addition of ice cubes. The immersions are at intervals of 30 seconds.[60] At the moment of immersion, a contraction can be noted, even if weak or inhibited by spasticity. The first response is strong, but successive immersion responses are weaker. The extensors are stimulated and the flexors are inhibited for about 20 minutes following the treatment. Some patients who have suffered hemiplegia begin to have voluntary control of muscles after only one ice water treatment, reacting strongly to the stimulation for about 10 minutes.[61]

Results of Cold: Depression, Stimulation, Derivation and Retrostasis

The application of cold to the body gives two effects: (1) the primary action of the cold, and (2) a secondary action or "reaction" to the cold. It is the secondary effects, or reaction, that are generally the most important in hydrotherapy, due to the reflexes that are set up in the internal organs as a result of the application of cold to the surface.[62]

An example of this principle is the following: If a cold compress is applied to the abdomen or back, the blood vessels of the pia mater over the brain, after a brief contraction, dilate widely and remain so for a long period. A warm compress applied to the feet or trunk, however, produces a *narrowing* of the vessels in the brain after a brief dilatation. This reaction of contracting vessels at a distance and dilating vessels locally, in this instance, the feet, is called *derivation*. Blood is actually transferred from the head to another part of the body.

In derivation, the blood comes to the surface mainly from the interior, about equally from all areas in the healthy body. If there are congested or inflamed organs or tissues, these areas will give up proportionately more blood than uninflamed parts. While any congested organ

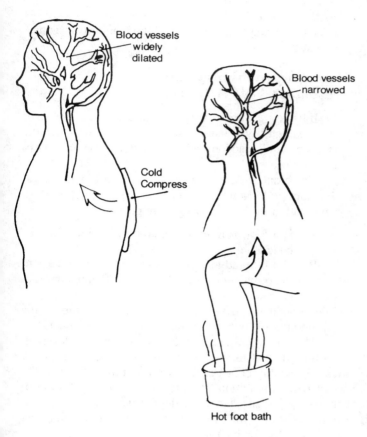

Hot foot bath

If cold compresses are applied to back or abdomen, blood vessels dilate inside the head. If a hot foot bath is used, the blood vessels inside the head get narrow, relieving pressure or congestion intracranially. Any congested or inflamed part will give up extra blood upon immersing the feet in hot water, thereby increasing the blood flow to and from the part. The improved circulation enhances healing processes.

will participate in this reaction, the internal blood vessel areas for which there is most use for this hydrostatic effect are chiefly the brain, the lungs, and the pelvic organs.

All hydrotherapeutic applications produce certain reflex effects. Heat, by its primary action, draws blood to

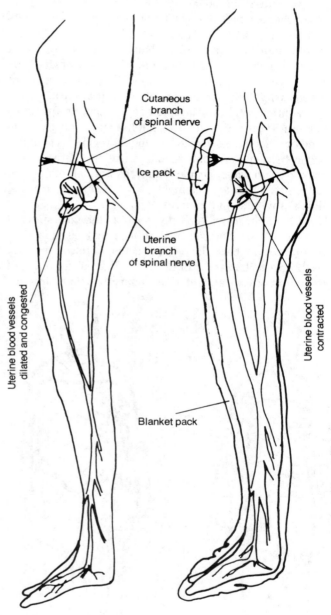

The most effective derivative is obtained by a combination of heat and cold as illustrated by this blanket pack to the hips and legs, and ice pack to the pelvis. The spinal nerves act through the skin receptors to mediate the reflex which contracts the blood vessels in the uterus, and dilates the blood vessels on the skin. The nerves supplying both the pelvic skin and the uterus enter the spinal cord at the same place, accounting for part of the vigor of the response.

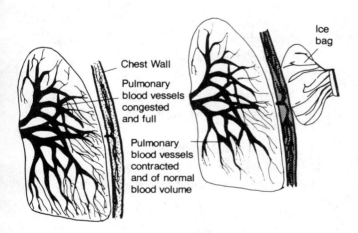

With the application of an ice bag to the chest wall, the congested pulmonary blood vessels contract, relieving the congestion through a process of derivation just as with heat.

the surface and may enhance this primary action by derivation. The primary action of cold is to drive blood to the interior, a process called *retrostasis*. The secondary or reflexive reaction to cold is to draw blood to the surface, which is termed *derivation* just as when produced by heat. A combination of primary and reflexive actions can be used to good advantage. For example, congestive headaches are relieved by the hot foot bath, together with cold compresses or ice bags to the head and neck. This combination is more effective than the derivative effect of the foot bath alone, although either portion of the combined treatment may be used alone if there is some reason why both phases cannot be used at once.

Acute pelvic inflammatory disease requires a vigorous derivative, such as a hot hip and leg pack, combined with ice bags to the suprapubic region. When preceded by a copious hot vaginal irrigation, the results in relief of pain usually come within the first ten minutes of the thirty minute treatment. The treatment can be finished with a cold mitten friction.

In certain forms of baths, such as the cool spray at 90°, the primary and secondary effects may be equal. In a prolonged cool bath, the primary action of retrostasis may be the greatest. A spray or needle bath at 60° for one-half minute may give a greater secondary reaction (drawing

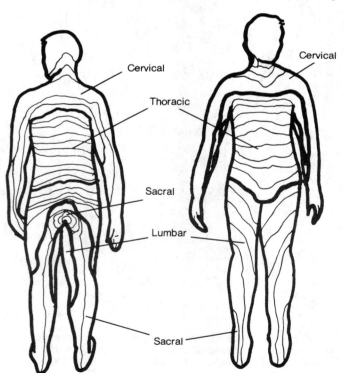

Cutaneous dermatomes. Applications to the skin in the various areas shown above have their primary and most intense reaction on the organs supplied by nerves that use the same spinal segment.

blood to the surface) than primary action. These reflex actions are brought about through the medium of the nervous system.

Summary of Primary and Secondary Cold Actions

If the application is very cold, under high pressure or accompanied by friction, and of short duration, the phenomena of reaction begin immediately when the application ceases.

Combinations of contraction from cold, and derivation from prolonged heat to another area are well used in combination in the following examples:

A. Hot foot bath and cool cloth to the forehead for headache.
B. Hot hip and leg pack combined with ice bags to the pubic area for acute pelvic inflammatory disease.

Cold applications have their greatest effect on the organs that lie nearest, but the distant effects are also useful.

The combined cross-section of all the capillaries of the body is 800 times that of the aorta (the major artery coming off the heart) and can profoundly influence the total body circulation. Prolonged or habitual chilling of the body has an adverse or depressive effect on repiration, digestion, muscle dexterity, circulation, phagocytosis, and biochemical reactions.

Primary Actions of Cold

1. When the application is local and not total body, contraction in the small blood vessels of the skin with dilatation of internal blood vessels after a brief contraction
2. Paleness of the skin because of less blood flow (The capillary blood pressure falls 6-11 mm. of mercury immediately.)
3. Gooseflesh and rough skin
4. Sensation of chilliness
5. Trembling, shivering, chattering of teeth
6. Pulse at first rapid, then slow
7. Respiration at first slow, then quick and gasping
8. Cooling of the skin
9. In most cases a slight rise of internal temperature
10. Perspiration checked
11. Initial retrostasis (driving blood to the interior)

Secondary Actions of Cold

1. With prolonged moderate cold applied to only a small area, dilatation of the small blood vessels of the surface and contraction of internal blood vessels: with total body cold surface contraction and deep dilatation when prolonged

2. Redness or blueness of skin (The capillary blood pressure rises in 5-8 minutes by 2-14 mm. A derivative effect is achieved as readily with cold as with heat.)

3. Soft skin, smooth and supple

4. Sensation of warmth

5. A sensation of comfort and sense of well-being

6. Slow pulse with increasing blood pressure

7. Respiration free, slower, and deeper

8. Slight warming of the skin

9. Fall of internal temperature

10. Increase of perspiration

11. Derivation (drawing blood from the interior) after 5-8 minutes to produce maximum possible dilatation of blood vessels in the skin

The Precapillary Sphincter

Of central importance to the reactions in hydrotherapy and massage is the precapillary sphincter. This most significant structure is a thickening of the muscular wall of the arteriole just before the take-off of the capillaries. It has a number of nerve feedbacks, motor and communication features which keep it in instant contact with the blood, nerves, and environment. The precapillary sphincter responds to temperature changes, hormones, mechanical stimuli such as stroking or percussion, drugs, certain classes of thoughts (embarrassment, fear, anger, and anxiety), tight clothing, and other factors. Its function is to control the blood flow to the capillaries and the blood pressure in the arteries.

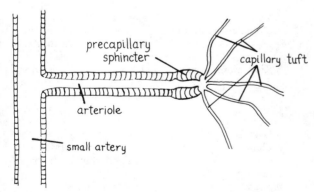

Precapillary Sphincter. The major anatomical structure for the control of circulation and blood pressure is the thickened muscle in the arteriole just before it gives rise to the "capillary tuft." By contracting or relaxing, the precapillary sphincter can control the flow of blood to the capillary bed. This sphincter is the most effective organ for the control of blood pressure. This muscle is sensitive to heat and cold, hormones, drugs, emotions, and mechanical factors such as pressure, friction, and percussion.

It is well-established that impressions made on the outside of the body affect the action of the organs within the body. Physical therapy is dependent upon this fundamental physiologic principle. While strong stimulation of any of the larger nerves in the body may cause changes in all the blood vessels throughout the vascular tree, these changes are most profound in those parts which have the most direct nerve connection with the part stimulated. For example, an ice bag applied over the stomach may cause a brief change in the size of the blood vessels of the brain, but the pronounced and more lasting changes are in the blood vessels of the stomach.[76]

For each internal organ there is a skin area which, when stimulated, causes a great change in the blood vessels of that organ. (See diagram in treatment technique section, Page 64). The nerves exercise a continual influence over the activities of the various internal organs. Their actions are accelerated, retarded, or even qualitatively changed through the influence of the nerves in the reflex arc.

There are several parts of the reflex mechanism. The purpose of the reflex arc is to transmit a signal for a pro-

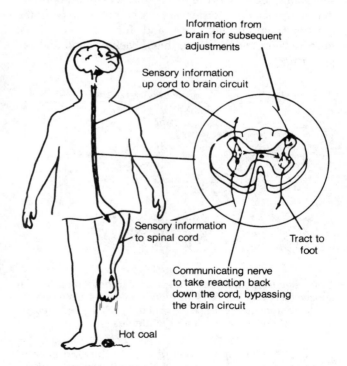

Reflex Arc. Actually both sides of the cord carry messages back down to the foot but only the right side is shown. Every sensory nerve in the body is in direct communication with every other nerve through the connections illustrated in this diagram—all the nerves to muscles, sweat glands, endocrine glands, salivary glands, blood vessels, etc. This mechanism is the most important single anatomical unit to mediate the effects of simple remedies.

tective action in the quickest way, without waiting for a message from the higher centers of the brain, which might be occupied with some interfering activity.

The Reflex Arc

1. A receptor organ: a sensing device to receive information about the environment

2. Afferent pathway: a nerve pathway to the interpreting center

3. An interpreting center: a center in the brain or spinal cord which acts to set up a series of reflexive activities which modify the status or activity of the effector organ (number 5 below)

4. Efferent pathway: a nerve pathway to the effector organ

5. An effector organ: muscles, blood vessels, precapillary sphincters, lymph channels, sweat glands, etc.

The nerve receptor organs are located in the skin. Sensors for heat and cold vary in number in different parts of the body; they are particularly sensitive to *changes* in temperature. They register either hot or cold sensations. Cold spots, special cold-sensitive points on the skin, listed in order are most numerous on the forehead, spine, leg, foot and forearm; and least numerous on the abdomen, thigh, back of hand and upper arm.[69]

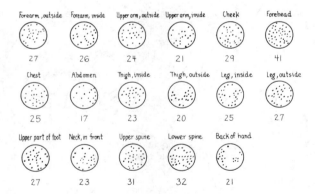

Cold receptors, skin. Some areas of skin have more thickly spaced receptors for cold sensation than others. Cold applications theoretically produce more benefit when used on areas where cold receptors are more numerous.

Whether the application of cold to the skin is *short and intense* or *long and moderate* will determine if the blood vessels in the underlying internal organs contract or dilate. Both reactions can be increased in degree by accompanying the cold application with friction pressure of about 15 to 35 pounds. The following areas are defined for the application of cold in order to obtain reactions in specific response areas:

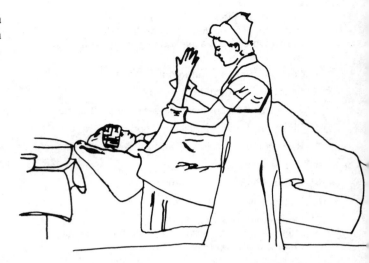

Cold Mitten Friction is an example of short and intense application of cold accompanied by friction usually generated at a force of between 15-35 pounds. This treatment is called a "tonic" treatment as it causes the blood vessels to contract. However, if ice is applied for several minutes, the blood vessels will dilate beginning usually after 4 to 6 minutes. The reaction is hastened by rubbing or percussion.

Area for Reaction	Where to Apply the Cold (or Hot) Applications
1. Brain	Head, neck, face, hands and feet, nasal mucous membranes
2. Face	Upper dorsal spine, hands, feet
3. Heart	The area over the heart (precordium), through the accelerator nerves (sympathetic)
4. Stomach and intestine	Lower dorsal spine, epigastrium, periumbilical region
5. Kidney and ureters	Lumbar and lower dorsal spine, lower portion of sternum, feet, skin of abdomen from navel to pubis
6. Bowels	Feet, abdomen
7. Bladder	Feet, lower abdomen, upper and inner thighs
8. Liver	Lower right chest
9. Spleen	Lower left chest
10. Upper respiratory tract	Hands, feet, upper chest
11. Pharynx and larynx	Skin of the neck
12. Lungs	Chest, thighs, upper dorsal region, shoulders, feet (especially soles)
13. Prostate, seminal vesicles, uterus, tubes and ovaries	Saddle area covered by the sitz bath

Area for Reaction	Where to Apply the Cold (or Hot) Applications
14. Uterus, tubes, ovaries and rectum	Lumbar region, abdomen, breasts, inner surface of thighs, feet, cervix uteri through the vagina (applications made to the cervix uteri are usually hot rather than cold), lower abdomen including the groin, and the upper inner surface of the thighs
15. All viscera	The skin immediately overlying the organ[272]

The application of cold to any area of the body (abdomen, soles, or legs) produces an immediate decrease in blood volume of the arm. An electric fan blowing over the nude body, especially if perspiring, produces powerful vasoconstriction (blood vessels narrow). The mere rattling of ice in a pan induces marked vasoconstriction in susceptible persons. The application of hot fomentations to the abdomen, the soles or legs, increases the arm volume,[65] meaning that the quantity of blood flowing into the arm has increased.

Water-drinking Reflex

The drinking of water at various temperatures produces interesting results in the arteries of the extremities. The mere act of swallowing causes the arm volume to decrease. Drinking either hot or cold water in some subjects causes peripheral vasoconstriction inducing a smaller volume of blood in the extremities.

Water drunk at 36° to 37.5° C. (97° to 100°) produces a decrease in blood volume. At 42° to 55° C. (107° to 132°) a definite decrease in arm volume occurs, and at 9° to 12° C. (48° to 54°) the most marked decrease of all. When the extremes of temperature are applied, either to the skin of the arm or leg, the soles of the feet, or to the abdomen in the area of the stomach, an alarm reaction occurs followed by constriction of blood vessels and a decrease in the volume of the arms.[67]

Persons who have just been exercising vigorously should not immediately drink either hot or cold drinks, as the blood flow to the extremities is thereby reduced and an extra burden of blood thrown into the vessels of the trunk. Persons whose deaths have been associated with vigorous exercise usually have had their first symptoms in the immediate post-exercise period, because they sit down immediately and drink a cool drink, either of which reduces circulation to the limbs and increases the volume of blood in the lungs, head, heart and liver; this imbalance of the circulation places a burden on the heart.

Temperature Extremes have Pronounced Effects

When heat treatments are given, the temperature should be raised slowly and steadily during the first 3-5 minutes. If advanced too rapidly, there is immediate vasoconstriction which may work against the objective of the treatment. Intense cold applied briefly to the skin of the face or head causes a reflexive dilatation of the blood vessels inside the head. Winternitz showed that prolonged moderate cold to the face and neck caused contraction of the blood vessels of the brain or other viscera reflexively connected with the overlying skin. Total body cold produces visceral artery dilatation, because of surface constriction, and reciprocal reflex dilatation. The skin contains unstriated muscle between the papillae and the fibrous tissue. When cold is applied, these unstriated muscles immediately squeeze the tissue, the capillaries lose their blood, and the lymphatics force their fluid

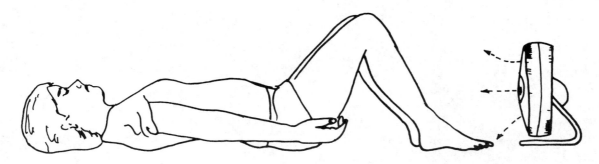

An electric fan blowing over the scantily-clad body, especially if perspiring or kept moist by sponging with tepid or cool water, causes a powerful constriction of the blood vessels in the extremities. A similar effect occurs with cold application to the soles, abdomen or legs. This treatment may be used in acute blood loss to transfer blood from the extremities to the more vital organs. In high blood pressure or impending stroke, use hot applications to the extremities, as the opposite reaction occurs with heat.

along their channels. When intense heat is applied, the same effect takes place.

Capillary constriction induced by cold lasts five to eight minutes after the removal of the cold, and the constriction is followed by dilatation so that the post-treatment diameter of the capillary is larger than before the application. The effect depends largely upon the duration of the stimulus with both hot and cold applications. The blood vessels will respond with their maximum peripheral dilatation in prolonged applications of cold. An ice bag left on for 20 minutes will cause maximum dilatation of skin blood vessels. This dilatation is the secondary effect, the primary constriction being produced by the initial stimulus during the first few minutes.

The initial 5 minute or more vasoconstriction in response to cold is produced by noradrenergic sympathetic vasomotor nerves. When a finger is placed in cold water, the constriction of blood vessels occurs first, followed by dilatation of blood vessels; but, interestingly there is a brief recurrence from time to time of constriction of blood vessels as long as the finger is kept in cold water, resulting in a pumping effect. The mechanism for dilatation of blood vessels in response to cold is not clear. It may be through the nerves, but could be through some biochemical substance, as the blood vessels will dilate in response to cold even when the nerves have been severed.[42]

Ice bags at 0° to 2° C. placed on the forehead decrease the temperature of the brain by 1.5°. An ice bag applied to the epigastrium produces an effect similar to sympathetic nerve stimulation by epinephrine, with lessened muscle tone of the stomach and irregular short but deep peristalic waves, accompanied by complete relaxation of the pylorus. When used for gastric and pyloric ulcers the pain relief can be dramatic. Applications to other areas of the body produce no such response in the stomach. This illustrates the principle that the major effect of temperature change of the skin is on the organs which lie immediately beneath the skin being treated.[68]

CHAPTER SEVEN

The Short Cold Bath

Benefits of the Short Cold Bath

The short cold bath is more useful and desirable in changing the functions of the body than any other form of therapeutics.[69] It should be utilized more frequently than it has been. It is the application of water to the body at temperatures varying from 90° down to 32° for one-half to three minutes with an average duration of one minute.

The common forms of cold baths are the wet hand rub, the mitten friction, the wet towel rub, the wet sheet rub, the needle bath, the shower spray, the percussion shower (douche), the full tub bath, the plunge, and the swimming bath. In all of these forms, application of cold water is made to all or to some particular part of the surface for only a brief time, the length of the treatment being determined by the condition of the patient, the degree of cold, and the size of the skin surface being treated. The effects of all these different forms of applying cold water to the body are essentially the same, varying mainly in intensity of reaction.

A better reaction comes from a combination of thermic and mechanical factors applied simultaneously as in the cold mitten friction, or the percussion shower. It is the cold in the water that achieves the effect on blood vessels, the water being simply a carrier for the cold, and the friction being a way to keep the cold more constantly in contact with the skin and to stimulate the nerves more vigorously.

After exposure to *mild,* sudden cold, the ability to perform muscular work increases![70] Use short cold baths for cancer, psychiatric disorders, shock, fever, hemorrhages, infections, and cerebral hemorrhage. Avoid prolonged chilling of large areas of the body in hyperthyroidism as that stimulates the thyroid. Avoid prolonged chilling in cancer as the stimulus to the thyroid can promote cancer growth. The short cold bath, however, benefits the cancer patient.[71]

Factors Determining the Responses to the Short Cold Bath

1. Ability of the individual to react. Kellogg stated that cold is intrinsically sedative, yet the primary effect (action) of cold is excitant, and the secondary effect (reaction) is "invigorating, restorative, tonic." The actual effect of cold depends upon the method of application, the area covered, the climate, the condition and susceptibility of the patient, and many other factors. A prolonged application of cold is at first excitant, then depressant, because of "fatigue" of the neuromuscular apparatus. One individual may react to a cold bath at a certain temperature as a stimulant, whereas another will react at the same temperature with a depressant action.[72]
2. Amount of skin surface involved in the application, a small skin surface area giving an *opposite effect* from total body treatments with cold.
3. Temperature of the water (the colder the water the greater the effect).
4. The quantity of water applied to the body at a single moment. The greater the mass of water, the greater the effect; as an example, a few jets of needle spray impinging against the body have less effect than 3 or 4 times the number of jets impinging.
5. The length of time of the application. Usually one minute is used, although as short an application as 30 seconds will be effective, and the treatment seldom goes beyond $3^1/_2$ minutes.
6. The mental attitude of the patient. If the treatment is feared or dreaded, the effect can be less desirable than if the patient has a relaxed attitude concerning the treatment.
7. The quality of skin over any organs. Sensory receptors are more numerous in some areas than others and a more brisk reaction can be expected. The skin

over an organ can be said to represent the organ beneath it for the purposes of obtaining a reaction.

8. The mechanical effects that accompany the applications. These mechanical effects include such things as massage, friction, and striking with a spray of water. They have the ability to augment the effect of the cold, by increasing the total amount of cold water that actually contacts the skin, and by increasing the sensory input from the area. This increases the summation of the impulses received in the interpreting center in the brain.

Reactions from Cold Baths

Because cold applied to the entire body depresses physiologic processes, inhibits perspiration and checks circulation to skin to reduce heat loss, the body at once receives sensory information that chilling is occurring by producing an alarm reaction through the central nervous system. By various adaptive processes the nervous system attempts to protect itself from depression of such a degree as to cause injury. The pituitary, thyroid, and adrenals are also brought into the act along with the blood vessels and nerves.

If, however, instead of becoming depressively chilled, the body remains in contact with cold water or cold air for only a brief time, its activities are heightened through these very adaptive processes instead of being slowed or depressed. The body reacts to depressant factors of chilling by *increasing* the force of the vital processes. To get into a cold bed when one is warm achieves this brief stimulation by cold. Short cold baths operate similarly. In this case the thermic impressions on the central nervous system are the important factor, not the transfer of heat. The body recognizes cold as a depressant action and counters immediately by increasing the vigor of the vital processes. The hemoglobin and white blood cells are both increased by this treatment.

The short cold bath also affects the pulse, the pulse pressure, and the blood pressure. In one study, sphygmographic tracings were done immediately before and after a short cold bath. Pulse tracings after the treatment showed a reduction in both rate and amplitude, illustrating the benefits of short cold baths on high blood pressure. It will be recognized that since the short cold bath diminishes the diastolic pressures an average of 12 points, and increases the systolic pressures an average of 18 points, the net result would increase pulse pressures by an average of 30 points. (The pulse pressure is the difference between the systolic and the diastolic readings.) Increasing the pulse pressure accelerates the circulation of the blood while decreasing the work load of the heart.

The cooler the bath the greater the reduction in pulse rate. The greater the area of the body exposed, the greater the reduction in the pulse. Whether or not friction accompanies the cool bath affects the degree of reduction in pulse rate.

To summarize the effects of the short cold bath on the arteries, we can say that it increases the tone of the heart and muscular walls of the arteries, which increases systolic blood pressure. The pulse rate, however, is diminished, the peripheral blood vessels are dilated, and the diastolic pressure decreases giving a salutary result in general circulation.

Cold Reflexes on Distant Systems

To put a foot or hand in a cold bath for five to ten minutes increases the number of both white and red blood cells in the blood stream. The short cold bath stimulates all the different functions of digestion, appetite, secretion of gastric juice, peristalsis, and colon emptying. The kidneys increase the quantity of urine as well as the quantity of total urinary solids, and the amount of urea excreted following a series of the baths.

Reflexive Influences of Cold

1. Contraction of arterial supply to the brain and nasal mucous membranes by prolonged chilling of the hands in cold water
2. Contraction of the arterial supply to the nasal mucous membranes by prolonged cold to the upper dorsal regions
3. Slowing of the heart rate with cold directly over the heart
4. Reduction in diameter of the heart with cold over the heart (up to one-half inch reduction shown by X-ray)
5. Reduction in thyroid activity with prolonged local applications on the neck
6. Contraction of the blood vessels of the stomach following epigastric cold
7. Reduction in gastric muscle tone and peristalsis with epigastric applications
8. Arterial contraction to the pelvic organs by brief and intense applications over the groin, low abdomen, and inner surface of the thighs
9. Contraction of the uterine muscles by prolonged cold sitz
10. Contraction of the cerebral arteries by applications to the face, forehead, scalp, and back of neck
11. Contraction of the arterial supply to the pharynx by applications to the sides of the neck just inferior to the angle of the jaw

General Indications for the Short Cold Bath

1. All chronic diseases where the bodily functions are below normal
2. Low vasomotor tone. (A cold bath is a heart tonic, one of the best. Congestive heart failure responds well in a receptive patient; begin with neutral water temperature and reduce the temperature two degrees with each subsequent bath.)
3. Hypothyroid conditions
4. Diabetes (aids in clearing the blood of excess sugar)
5. Obesity
6. Skin diseases
7. Infections: malaria, epididymitis and prostatitis, salpingitis, abscesses, and carbuncles[73]
8. Any disorder for which a fever treatment is indicated but the condition of the patient or circumstances preclude its use
9. Scarlet fever[74] [75]

Contraindications for Short Cold Bath

1. Cold person.
2. Excessive fatigue.
3. Suspected shock or collapse.
4. Poor kidney function. There is a close relationship between the kidneys and the skin. In advanced diseases of the kidneys with a reduction in function the skin also becomes sluggish in performing its functions and cannot react as usually expected.
5. Cardiovascular disease. Use caution in advanced cardiovascular disease and arteriosclerosis because of the expected increase in systolic blood pressure with cold applications.
6. Hyperthyroidism. The basal metabolic rate (BMR) is further increased.

Functional Results of Short Cold Applications

1. Stimulation of mental activity with applications to face and head
2. Increase in respiratory rate with applications to chest, or to the skin generally, followed by deeper, slower respirations
3. Increase in heart rate and cardiac output can be enhanced by slapping the chest with cold towels

4. Dilatation of blood vessels to an internal organ following short, intense, cold percussion shower (douche) to the corresponding reflex area (Example: a short, cold, percussion shower to the sacrum or feet dilates the uterine arteries)
5. Contraction of the muscles of the bladder, the bowels, and the uterus by short cold applications to the abdomen, hands or feet
6. Dilatation of arteries to the liver by short, cold applications over the liver
7. Increased gastric secretion by moderately prolonged, cold applications to the epigastrium
8. Increased free and total hydrochloric acid by cold to the abdominal walls and thighs
9. General constriction of the skin blood vessels when the surface of the body is chilled, demonstrating the importance of proper dress in equalizing the circulation

An important principle to be remembered in giving the short cold bath, as in most other treatments, is that extremes in temperature may cause a very intense reaction initially in an opposite direction from the one desired. Thus, applications that are extremely hot or extremely cold (ice) may be detrimental, or less effective, than those at milder temperatures, the exception, of course, being when a drastic reaction is needed, as to stop hemorrhage in nosebleed, or postpartum bleeding.[264]

Summary of Benefits of the Short Cold Bath

A. The pulse is increased. The pulse pressure increases an average of 30 points which increases the circulation of the blood. This is brought about by an average increase in the systolic blood pressure of 18 points and an average decrease of 12 points in the diastolic.
B. Neuromuscular transmission is made more effective.
C. Respiration increases.
D. Muscles increase in tone and elasticity; work capacity increases, fatigue decreases.
E. The skin is toned up.
F. Basal metabolic rate and thyroid function increase.
G. Hemoglobin, red blood cells and white blood cells all increase.
H. Urine production increases.
I. Constipation is relieved.

CHAPTER EIGHT

Hot Applications

General Features

The application of intense heat is initially an excitant and then decidedly a depressant. Heat contracts yellow elastic tissue, but relaxes the white fibrous tissue of ligaments and tendons. The vascular dilatation due to heat is passive; that due to cold is active. When the vessels of one area supplied by an artery are dilated, the vessels in the remaining portions of that same artery as well as other arteries at a distance may be contracted. Increased blood in one area gives rise to a compensatory blood reduction in a correlated blood pressure area. This explains the pain relief given by applying heat to an arthritic joint or over a congested nerve or muscle. As the blood vessels in the inflamed area contract, the tension in the tissues is relieved, and pain abates. The same effect occurs with the relief of internal pain which results from a general hot application.

Hot applications of any kind lower the alkalinity locally of the blood in that part. It should be emphasized, therefore, to finish every hot application with a cold application of some sort, the cold serving to reinstate normal alkalinity of the blood and increase resistance to accidental exposure to chilling.

Hot air hinders gas exchange in the lungs and causes an increase in the rate of breathing, but produces shallow breathing. Heat and moisture to the point of saturation interfere with the elimination of wastes through the lungs. If the air in the treatment room becomes heavy with fog it produces pulmonary water saturation which interferes with pulmonary exchange. The pulse rate goes up as the temperature of the room air or the bath goes up.

Because of an increase in respiration with a hot bath, alkaline substances in the blood are excreted by the kidneys, causing a rise in urinary pH. The diuresis seen with baths is an effect produced by the bath, more or less independent of the temperature used.

Specific Reactions to Hot Applications

1. Prolonged hot applications to the reflex areas of the skin produce passive dilatation of blood vessels in the corresponding organ.
2. Applications to the chest increase expectoration and respiration.
3. Reduction in blood pressure and cardiac output, but increase in force of heart beat is produced by long, hot applications over the heart.
4. Increased gastric secretion and motility by hot applications over the stomach after meals results in more rapid digestion. if applied before meals, hot applications decrease tone and secondary gastric secretions, which can decrease nausea or pain in the stomach.
5. Heat at 125° to the epigastrium causes effects like parasympathetic stimulation, with increased tone of the muscles in a relaxed stomach, and decreased tone

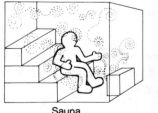
Sauna

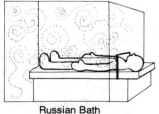
Russian Bath

The Russian bath has an advantage over the sauna in that the head is kept out of the steam room. The person can breathe cool, dry air, and the head can be kept cool. Both heat and moisture in air hinder pulmonary gas exchange, and interfere with the elimination of water and wastes through the lungs.

in a contracted stomach. Peristalsis under the influence of this heat is altered to increase the opening of the pylorus. These effects are not secured by heat to other areas and thus are specific for the skin of the epigastrium.

6. Prolonged hot applications to the abdomen lessen intestinal peristalsis in diarrhea and colic, and increase motility in ileus (intestinal paralysis).
7. Prolonged hot applications to the pelvis, as a fomentation, pack or sitz bath, relax the muscles of the bladder, the rectum and the uterus, dilate their blood vessels and increase the menstrual flow.
8. A large application to the trunk, as a hot trunk pack in biliary or renal colic, relaxes the muscles of the bile ducts, the gallbladder or the ureters, and aids in relieving the pain due to spasm in these hollow organs.
9. Mild heat stimulation of the areas over the colon produces efforts at expulsion of feces from the colon and more rapid emptying of the ileum into the colon.
10. Stimulation by heat or a mustard plaster over the abdomen from the navel to the pubic bone, or over the kidneys at the back causes an increased production of urine with decreased specific gravity lasting about an hour.

Physiologic Mechanisms Making Hydrotherapy Effective

1. There is something related to a placebo effect in hydrotherapy which should be fully exploited in all stages of pain or discomfort. Apparently the brain makes a "comfort" hormone (endorphins) upon the application of a placebo.
2. The removal of toxins from the body follows certain conditions such as diaphoresis, an increase in white blood cells, and an increase in circulation.
3. Dilation of blood vessels or constriction can be accomplished by the intensity of the heat and the direction of the flow of the heat, whether the temperature is being raised or lowered.
4. The laying on of hands can be quite beneficial as many sick patients will attest. It can be speculated that the mechanism is through the flow of heat or even of electrons. Perhaps a "comfort" hormone is produced as in item one above.
5. Following the application of hydrotherapy the antibacterial lysozymes become more effective in fighting bacteria, because of the increased heat and a decrease in pH. These lysozymes are produced in the nasal secretions and other body fluids.
6. There can be a balancing of the circulation by the use of hydrotherapy.

7. The "gate mechanism" may be the explanation as to how hydrotherapy is effective in the treatment of pain. This mechanism has to do with the interference of certain nerve impulses if other impulses are competing for the use of the "gate." Pain-temperature pathways are close together in the long spinal tracts. Communicating pathways in the spinal cord are very numerous. It may be that much traffic on the pain pathways becomes impeded by similar traffic on the nearby temperature pathways.

Favorable and Unfavorable Effects in Using Heat

1. Exercise sufficient to warm the body promotes a reaction. This is true whether the exercise is taken before or after a heat treatment. It should be kept in mind in exercising individuals, however, that very heavy and prolonged exercise to the point of causing muscular tenderness can produce albuminuria, cylindruria, hematuria, and a reduction in glomerular filtration rate. These can be recognized by dark and scanty urine, sometimes dark reddish brown. It is a benign condition which reverses itself after several days. It may be called pseudonephritis. However, since dehydration also occurs with some heat treatments, if dehydration should occur with the exercise, the kidneys might fail to maintain the blood pH during the bath. Therefore, the patient who complains of sore muscles from exercising must be given plenty of water before a heat treatment; adequate kidney function in these cases can be assessed by urinalysis.
2. Fatigue is not conducive to a prompt and vigorous reaction.
3. Infants and old people or those of low vitality can be expected to react poorly. General good physical condition enhances reaction.
4. A chilled patient may react slowly, feebly, or not at all. Start all treatments with a warm patient, even if you must give a hot foot bath or dry blanket pack beforehand.
5. Interactions between therapist and patient can influence the effectiveness of the treatment. There should be no contention, no levity, no formality, or tense shyness. Move easily, quietly, and without a show of haste or hint of delay.
6. Disorderliness of the room can offend the sensibilities of some patients and interfere with reaction. Noisy footsteps or constantly humming equipment may be distracting. There should be no interruptions during treatments except for urgent matters.
7. Friction or percussion may increase the ability of the patient to react.

8. If a cold mitten friction is started while the last fomentation is still in place and the hot foot bath is being continued, a better reaction is generally produced.
9. The effectiveness of hydrotherapy is probably diminished by eating just before or just after a treatment, or by the heavy use of sugar and oil, by most drugs, and by alcohol.
10. The blood vessels of the skin, the lymphatic vessels, the millions of nerve endings, the fixed tissue macrophages, the vasculature of the hair follicles, the detoxification potential of the sweat glands, and a number of other factors unite to make the skin very effective in the treatment of disease. When the skin is working perfectly, such organs as the heart, the liver, the kidneys, and the gastrointestinal tract are protected to some degree from overwork. It has been shown that the sweat glands are likely to become diseased when there is long-standing kidney disease. This condition results from the overuse of the sweat glands to excrete the toxic wastes ordinarily excreted by the kidneys.
11. Hydrotherapy brings boils to a head by softening the skin causing the path of least resistance to be toward the skin rather than toward the deeper tissues.
12. Even in very vascular tissues, the moist heat of a poultice or fomentation may penetrate the tissues and muscles to a depth of over 20 millimeters, and in some instances up to 75 millimeters. Dry applications do not generally heat the tissues as effectively.
13. Hydrotherapy increases the sense of well-being and relaxation.
14. The pumping action of alternating hot and cold hydrotherapy procedures tends to carry away toxins and bring in nutrients.
15. Heat applied to the skin of the abdominal wall of normal humans inhibits motor activity of the stomach, small bowel and colon. Cold to the skin of the abdomen, however, stimulates tonus and peristaltic activity. Drinking hot or cold water reverses these responses. Cold applied to the abdominal walls and thighs increases both free and hydrochloric acid![76]

Educating the Temperature Adjustment Mechanisms

The body is marvelously adapted to take care of the necessary temperature adjustments of the individual. Our Creator has provided delicate structures in the skin which sense temperature changes. They are probably the naked nerve endings that sense not only the actual temperature, but also the amount and rate of the change of skin temperature as well as the direction which the skin temperature is changing, whether up or down. Thus, the central nervous system is provided with information which causes the skin to be reflexively regulated by many responses to prevent the loss or accumulation of heat. The deep structures of the body are similarly provided with sensory mechanisms which are sensitive to heat and cold, predominantly in the heart and pulmonary circulations, the great veins near the heart, and the spinal cord, as well as in the anterior hypothalamus.

It is well known that individuals who move to cold climates quickly adjust to the cold. The same can be said of those moving to the tropics. This process is called acclimatization. It occurs also in response to the clothing one wears and to certain life style factors as the use of hot or cool baths, air conditioners, saunas, and similar factors.

The electric light box achieves an air heat from 140° to 165°. The hot air dilates the blood vessels in the skin and draws blood to the surface of the body. With heat treatments of any kind as much as 60% of the blood can be held in the peripheral blood vessels.[77] When the temperature of the skin is quickly reversed as by alternating the light treatment with a cold shower, an active response occurs in the vascular network in the skin and provides a more rapid exchange of blood. Subsequent treatments show an apparent "education" of the adaptive mechanisms with enhancement of the response and a sense of well-being much appreciated by the average patient. This has been called an educational bath, because it develops a responsiveness in these physiologic mechanisms, a responsiveness that may be sluggish in the chronically ill or poorly acclimatized person. Repeated hot and cold baths as well as exercise and good health habits improve the ability of the adaptive and eliminative functions to induce healing.

Right and Left Sides React Together

A further marvel of the fine adjustments of the temperature regulating mechanism is the provision for a sympathetic response of one hand when the opposite hand is chilled or heated, and the hands when the feet are chilled or heated, and the same for the feet when the hands are chilled or heated.[78] The contralateral response occurs in as little as one second! Heating the legs will cause reflexive vasodilatation elsewhere in the body with a latency of only 10 to 15 seconds. The sweat glands themselves produce bradykinin, a substance which causes vasodilatation in the very region of sweating.[91] The fine detail of functional design denotes the caretaking of Divine Intelligence. Bradykinin is a potent vasodilator, acting directly on blood vessels. It is possible that with generalized body heating bradykinin would be released everywhere to dilate blood vessels all over the body. It may be this action that causes the sensation of fainting in an individual rising from a bath following a fever treatment.

Another Method of Stimulating the Skin

Vasomotor excitation following mechanical stimulation of the skin may be very powerful, approaching that of the application of heat or cold. Friction and percussion are the two major methods of applying mechanical stimulation. Both friction and percussion may be applied by the hand, by a mechanical device, or by delivering a stream of water at varying pressures. Three grades of friction are recognized as follows:

1. *Light friction* which causes a rise in blood pressure, increased pulse rate, and increased respiratory rate. There is contraction of small blood vessels with very light friction which may persist for several hours. The lightest touch possible with the fingernails in a scratching action on the skin can be helpful in driving blood internally in cases of hemorrhage to make the blood available for the vital centers. The skin should be frictioned only once in hemorrhage and care should be exercised that the scratching does not result in a red mark, indicating vasodilation.

2. *Energetic friction* which causes at first a pronounced contraction of blood vessels, quickly followed by dilatation of surface vessels, and reduction in body temperature by several tenths of a degree. In a debilitated patient this treatment may be used to reduce fever.

3. *Very vigorous friction* which produces a wide dilatation of blood vessels, slowing of the heart and respiration, and a great increase in heat elimination, so that the temperature may fall as much as one or two degrees. This treatment may be used in strong, young patients to reduce fever.

COMPARISON OF MAJOR RESPONSES OF COLD AND HEAT

	Cold	Heat
General Effects	Primary: excitant after initial depressant	Primary: excitant if intense
	Short applications: excitant by tonic reaction	Short: depressant by atonic reaction
	Prolonged applications: depressant by the influence on the metabolic function	Prolonged: mixed, excitant and depressant
Special Effects	Heart: first fast, then slow	Heart: first slow, then fast
	Vessels: the action, contraction; the reaction, dilatation	Vessels: the action, dilatation; the reaction, contraction when intense
	Nerves: benumbs	Nerves: excites
	Muscles: reduces volume	Muscles: increases volume
	Respiration: slows and deepens	Respiration: quickens
	Stomach: increases hydrochloric acid and motion	Stomach: decreases hydrochloric acid and motion
	Blood: increases blood count, both RBC's (30 to 50%) and WBC's (15-150%); increases phagocytosis unless prolonged to chilling	Blood: increases blood count, both RBC's and WBC's; increases phagocytosis
	Kidneys: congests and stimulates	Kidneys: reduces activity
	Metabolism: increases CO_2 in blood by increasing production of CO_2; decreases urea; improves oxidation	Metabolism: decreases CO_2 in the blood by overbreathing; increases urea and general protein wastes

Measured in Angstrom units

	$\frac{1}{10,000}$
	$\frac{1}{1,000}$
Gamma Rays Emitted By Radioactive Substances	$\frac{1}{100}$
	$\frac{1}{10}$
	1
	10
	100
Ultraviolet Rays	1,000
	10,000
	100,000
Infrared Rays	1,000,000

Man-made rays used in medical diagnoses and treatments

Visible Light

Measured in Meters

	$\frac{1}{1,000}$
	$\frac{1}{100}$
	$\frac{1}{10}$
	1
	10
	100
	1,000
	10,000
	100,000
Electric Waves	1,000,000
	10,000,000
60 Cycle A C	100,000,000

Microwave (Radar)

Television

Communications

The electromagnetic spectrum.

Sunshine

Sunlight causes a very powerful reaction in the skin which develops pigment. Certain individuals are genetically fashioned with fair skin so that they are unable to respond satisfactorily to protect the skin from too much sunlight by bringing pigment to the surface. These individuals, albinos, and other extensively depigmented persons (those having vitiligo and related disorders) should not have prolonged exposure to sunlight.

It is noteworthy that the very young and the very old tolerate sunlight better than those in the childbearing years, and are less likely to get dangerous or painful burns. This characteristic apparently has to do with hormone function.

There are some diseases (such as lupus erythematosus and bullous pemphigus) that may be made worse by much exposure to sunlight. Nevertheless, very small or moderate exposure even in these cases may be beneficial, perhaps five to ten minutes daily on each side of the body. The utmost care must be exercised, however, that the patient's condition is not made worse. It may be well to start with putting the patient fully clothed outdoors in deep or partial shade for five to ten minutes. Then progress to a few seconds of walking in the sun. Then expose an extremity, and so forth.

Systemic Effects of Temperature Changes

Altering the body temperature by means of steam in a chamber at 80° to 120° has been found to significantly increase the mean heart rate (62%), the serum growth hormone (142%), and the plasma renin activity (95%). One hour after a 20 to 40 minute sauna the growth hormone has returned to control levels, but the renin activity still remains higher than before the bath. Urinary sodium excretion decreases by 46% during the first six hour period from the beginning of the sauna bath.[79]

Electromagnetic scale. The human body cannot sense electromagnetic waves except for the single octave of visible light and the heat waves. The shortest waves are the gamma rays measuring from 0.5 to 0.06 Angstrom units (A.U.). An A.U. is one ten millionth of a millimeter. The longest waves are the Hertzian rays which are in the neighborhood of 4 inches to 100,000 miles in length, with 100 to 300 miles being commonest. Their vibration frequency is from millions to merely thousands of vibrations per second. The intensity of radiation varies inversely as the square of the distance from the wave source. Even a short distance back from a wave source will greatly reduce the effective radiation received. Increasing the distance between the radiation source and the object by a factor of two decreases the intensity of radiation received on the object by 4 times!

Because of certain research done with animals, it is felt best not to raise the body temperature of pregnant women. Guinea pigs at all stages of gestation were exposed to temperatures of 42° to 43° C. for one hour daily on certain days after pregnancy began (1, 2, 4, or 8 days). High doses of heat stress caused maternal death, smaller doses caused fetal death, even smaller doses caused abortion, lesser levels produced fetal malformations, and very small temperature elevations caused no effect. The fetal abnormalities were microcephaly, hypoplasia of digits, umbilical hernia, clubfoot, and arthrogryposis.[80]

Because of this animal research and a retrospective study done in humans, we suggest the possible contraindication to the use of fever treatment in pregnant women during the first three months of pregnancy, at the time of anterior neural-groove closure. In a review of 63 pregnancies investigating anencephalic infants, seven of the 63 pregnancies (11%) had a history of maternal fever near the presumed time of closure of the neural-groove. Five had fever with temperatures ranging from 38.9° to 40° C. (103° to 104.6°). Two had sauna baths at about the same period of gestation, with no infectious agent present.[81]

Chilling animals causes the blood sugar to rise as the blood sugar is related to glycogenolysis in the liver resulting in a high hepatic glucose output. In the chilled animal, probably because of a combination of the glycogenolysis factor and decreased peripheral glucose utilization in chilled tissues, the plasma glucose level climbs. Hypothermia has been used in various surgical procedures and is associated with a decrease in tissue oxygen consumption. Hypothermia interferes with the action of insulin in animals. A contributing factor in the elevation of blood sugar is the release of adrenalin in the chilled animal which results in the greater release of glucose by the liver.[82]

Mammals reduce the heat in the head by breathing cool air across the resonant cavity of the head, the sinuses, and the nasal cavities. As the blood transfers its warmth to the air flowing through the nasal passages which are rich in blood vessels, the blood is cooled, both going to and coming from the brain. This cooling action is one very good reason why a jogger or one who is working vigorously should breathe through the nose, in order to keep the mucous membranes on the under surface of the cranium cool. Some cooling comes from the oral cavity, but more from the nasal mucous membranes. Because the nasal and sinus cavities are not cooled thereby, breathing hot air is not the most conducive to health, either mental or physical.[83]

An interesting temperature sensation occurs in baths. If the patient enters the bath at 37.5° C., the bath water is above the normal skin temperature and the patient initially feels warm. After a short while, he feels only com-

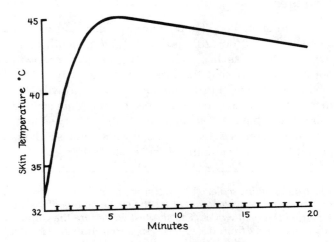

Exercise produces a large, brief increase in blood flow to a part; hot packs cause a smaller flow but it is more prolonged and results in a greater total increase in the circulation. The reaction of the circulation is related to the intensity of the heat and the duration of the application. After 7 minutes of hot packs the flow of blood reaches its peak, then falls off slightly during the next 20 minutes, even if the temperature remains constant. At about 7 minutes the skin temperature reaches its height (45.4° C.) Ref. Physical Therapy 52:273-8 March 1972.

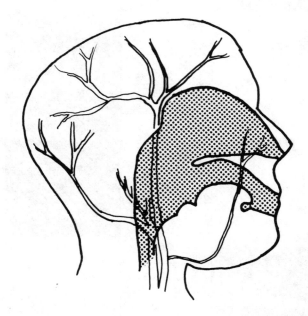

Breathing through the nose is especially important when the blood is being heated, as with exercise or heating treatments. Arterial blood going to the brain is cooled by its passage near and through the nasal passages, which are cooled by air and evaporation.

fortable, and usually later feels somewhat cooler than comfortable. For a patient who was kept for days in a neutral bath as a control, it was found that the subject felt comfortable only when the temperature of the water was sufficient to cause a slight fever. Symptoms experienced by various subjects in prolonged neutral baths include dyspnea, palpitation, noticable pulsation in the extremities, mental symptoms (excitability, easy loss of temper, inability to think of right words, and faintness). These mental symptoms are relieved by inhaling oxygen or CO_2. Occasionally tetany has been seen, starting usually with tonic spasms of the muscles of the hands.

CHAPTER NINE

The Marvels of Water

Water

Water as a remedial agent is unsurpassed, approaching that of a universal remedy in its various applications of steam, hot water, cold water and ice. It can be used successfully in more areas than any other remedy. Its very abundance, availability, economy and ease of application make it one of the blessings of heaven for application as a simple and rational remedy. It is the universal solvent, non-irritating, and specially designed by the Creator for use in healing. It is able to give up its heat rapidly, but does not cool too rapidly for convenience. It has a high heat capacity and a high latent heat capacity with change of state. Its viscosity is perfect for easy use. It has the proper density for buoyancy when total body

baths are used. It is reassuring to contemplate that a loving and all-wise Creator provided water for our needs before He placed us on this planet, just as our cleansing from the results of sin was provided before there was a need.

Latent Heat of Freezing

When one gram of ice at 0° C. changes to 1 gram of water also at 0° C. a certain amount of energy is required. This energy is stored in the water at the time of the changing from ice to water, and is given up when the water changes from the liquid form to the solid form. This is called *latent heat*. Explained in another way, to change ice to water requires energy which is stored in the water.

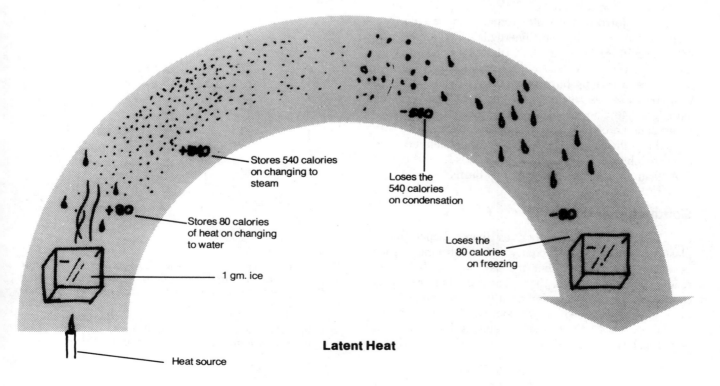

Stores 540 calories on changing to steam

Loses the 540 calories on condensation

Stores 80 calories of heat on changing to water

1 gm. ice

Loses the 80 calories on freezing

Heat source

Latent Heat

If ice at 1° C. is changed to water at 1° C. approximately 80 calories of heat will be stored in the water, yet no change in recorded temperature can be detected by a thermometer .

Another important feature of the ability of water to absorb heat is discovered when comparing water with other fluids. If liquid mercury is used to transfer heat to water, the mercury will have to lose 30° C. in order to raise the temperature of water only 1° C! These features of water physics determine its usefulness in administering the simple remedies. We can only marvel at the millions of tiny bits of evidence everywhere we look that unite in a grand symphony to declare the Creator's infinitely complex and painstaking design. The careless glance does not reveal the sublime omniscience. But to the reverent eye the things of nature—no less than the deepest and tenderest earthly ties that human hearts can know—reveal that every act of the Divine Hand is an act of benevolent graciousness.

Latent Heat of Vaporization

To change one gram of liquid water to one gram of water vapor at the same temperature of 100° C. requires approximately 540 calories, stored in the water vapor. This amount of energy is required to change the form of water from liquid to vapor. Although there is no change in external temperature of the water as it changes from liquid form at 100° C. to vapor form at 100° C., this heat is stored in the vapor. Approximately one calorie is required to change water at 90° C. to water at 91° C., but to change the *form* of the water requires much energy to disperse the molecules. This energy is called *latent heat of vaporization*. As water cools from water vapor to liquid water, the latent heat of vaporization is given up. Therefore, a serious burn may occur if water vapor (a gas) condenses as steam (small liquid particles) on the skin. The 540 calories which were stored at the time of vaporization are given up to the environment, in this case the skin, at the time of condensation. This latent heat can cause much injury to sensitive tissues. It is for this reason that steam injuries are often serious burns.

Conduction of Heat

Certain substances (such as wood, paper, cloth, plastic, etc.) conduct heat poorly. Other substances (such as water, silver, and other metals) conduct heat very readily. For this reason, these materials that are highly conductive feel colder or hotter at the same temperature than do substances which are poor conductors of heat.

Water has 27 times greater capacity for conducting heat than has air. Therefore, one can step into a refrigera-

tor at 32° with the skin bare and suffer little discomfort. If, however, one stepped into a tub of water at 32° he would feel a shock because of the much greater ability of water to conduct heat from the surface of the body. This property of massive conduction of temperature makes water very valuable in applying thermic stimuli to the skin surface.

Since water is a good conductor, there is marked cooling of the body by an ice rub because actual heat transfers from the body to the ice, being stored in the melted water as latent heat. The same thing occurs in the wet sheet pack with evaporation, since heat is transferred from the body to the water as it vaporizes from the surface of the body, giving off approximately 540 calories per gram of vapor produced. For this reason, it is rarely necessary to use ice, since water in evaporation carries away large quantities of heat from the body.

Physical Properties of Water

In order to apply hydrotherapy in the most intelligent way, it is necessary to be knowledgeable about the theories involved in the use of water. Water possesses physical and chemical properties that make it ideal for the transfer of heat. It should be kept in mind that water is merely the agent to conduct heat. Profound changes in the physiology of the body can be produced by shifting the amount of heat only a few degrees up or down. The important thing to understand is that water has great heat-conveying and tactile properties which cause pronounced

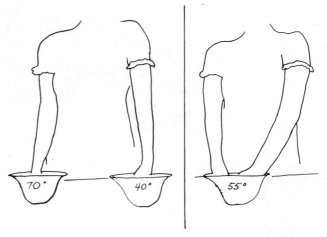

If at first one hand is placed in water at 70° and the other at 40°, then after the hands have become accustomed to the water temperature, both hands are removed and placed in a single basin at 55°, the water will feel cold to one hand and warm to the other. This illustrates the principle that a change in temperature is appreciated more keenly by the nerves than the actual temperature of the environment.

effects on the vascular system, the nervous system, the muscles, the metabolism, white blood cells, immune system, endocrines, and other tissues and organs.

The sensory receptors are more keenly aware of temperature changes than of absolute temperature. To illustrate, the hands may be placed in water, one hand in water at 70°, the other hand in water at 40°. If, after allowing the hand to become accustomed to the water temperature, both hands are removed and placed in a single basin containing water at 55°, one hand will sense the water as cold, the other hand will sense the water as hot, although both hands are in the same pan of water. The thermic impression is due to the *change* in temperature, in one instance from very cold to *less cold* and in the other instance from slightly warm to *less warm*.

If mechanical stimulation is given to the skin along with the temperature changes, a greater impression can be made on the nervous system. With mechanical stimulation, such as percussion from streams of water, rubbing or brushing of the skin during the application of hot or cold water, more water can be brought against the skin at any one moment, thus decidedly changing the skin temperature. At the same time, the mechanical stimulation, apart from the temperature change, evokes a vascular, nervous, or muscular response.

Because of the distribution of heat by means of the blood circulation, there is not a great penetration of heat from a hot fomentation or a locally applied bath, to the surrounding tissues. As the heat from the fomentation passes into the body, the blood is constantly removing much of the heat, preventing a great build up of heat in the deeper tissues. Deep internal organs are *more influenced* by local applications of heat *through reflexive effects than by local heating.*

CHAPTER TEN

How To Use Water To Treat Illness

Introduction

To successfully work with a sick person, the medical missionary should first learn to be quiet, quick, and efficient. Success in applying the physiologic stimuli as simple remedies depends on attention to small details. This point cannot be overemphasized. Carefulness for the comfort, safety, and proper functioning of each organ will be repaid in success in the treatment of disease.

Study the disposition of the patient and know when to talk and when to remain silent. Very sick people usually prefer to remain silent, since conversation requires a great deal of emotional and mental energy. Do not, however, become withdrawn and cheerless. Avoid talking about other sick cases that you know, either with the patient or with others in the presence of the patient. Remain hopeful and quietly cheerful. It is the duty of every person who attends the sick, from the minister to the physician, to keep the room pleasant, neat, orderly, properly ventilated and as comfortably quiet as possible.

The bed should be changed daily for a very sick patient and kept smooth and fresh. Spills and soils on the sheets can be covered with a towel or disposable paper. The nurse should not always be busying around as the bustle wearies the patient. Even touching the bed may be disturbing, and rubbing the bed or the patient in a monotonous way may interfere with the relaxation of the patient. It is the nurse's duty to see that visitors do not jostle the bed or weary the patient.

Use a flexible straw for drinking. Take axillary rather than oral temperatures wherever possible to avoid needless errors occasioned by talking, drinking, eating or sleeping with the mouth open. Remember that the patient's afternoon temperature is almost always higher than the morning reading. Do not awaken a patient out of sleep for routine procedures unless unusually urgent. Never allow a patient to have cold hands or feet. Never give cold treatments when the patient is either chilly or perspiring. Never touch a patient with cold hands.

Always give the patient a sense of fastidious cleanliness without being fussy. Never speak in a conciliatory or babyish voice to a patient. Avoid using the plural first person for the singular second person, such as "Let us now drink our water." Never tease a patient or engage in the slightest hint of frivolity. Never criticize the physician or another helper in the patient's case. Do not burden the patient by relating even the slightest trouble in your own family or that of mutual friends. Avoid any "heavy" subject.

Be alert to the spiritual needs of the patient, and at the proper time minister efficiently to these needs. Refrain altogether from expressing any religious view which might conflict with the religious views held by the patient. There is much that is wholesome and positive to be drawn from the Holy Scriptures without dealing with the controversial or negative at a time of physical stress. You may properly allow the patient to see your own genuine religious faith. Many times this manifestation of calm trust in God will decide the case favorably. The confidence of the nurse, doctor, or attendant in unseen agencies, and his faith that his prayers in behalf of the patient will be heard, will give confidence, and balance the mind of the one who is passing through the crisis.

Tender, Loving Carefulness

1. Have the room warm and free of drafts.
2. No overhead light should shine in the patient's eyes.
3. Cover furniture, rugs, bedding, and other objects that may be water damaged during the treatment.

4. Avoid radios, tape recorders, and all distracting noise.
5. Plan ahead and assemble all necessary articles.
6. Stay with the patient, or within easy calling distance.
7. Don't be too talkative.
8. Constantly observe the effects of the treatment.
9. Make your changes quickly, but do not appear to rush.
10. Be neat and orderly as you work.
11. Be economical of time, linen, etc.
12. Explain the procedures, quietly announcing what is coming next and what effect is desired.
13. When using a heating treatment, put a cold compress to the head or neck when the patient begins to sweat, or when the oral temperature reaches 100°. Do not apply the cold to the head too early, or the desired reaction may be aborted. Do not delay too long or the patient may get congestion of the head.
14. Allow no unnecessary exposure; uncover only the part under immediate treatment.
15. The patient should be comfortable at all times. Protect from burns, falling, uncomfortable positions, etc. No treatment should be torture.
16. Avoid chilling. Remember that the "reaction time" after the treatment is an essential part of the treatment. Put the patient to bed for 30-60 minutes to accomplish this part.

When fomentations are first applied, they are made more tolerable by gently wiping the area with the bare hand as often as necessary. This wipes away the moisture which serves as a conductor of heat.

Baths

1. Cataract shower, jet shower, pail pour shower bath, spray douche. Water is poured from overhead or delivered under pressure from an ordinary bathroom shower or a garden hose adding mechanical stimulation to the effect of the water temperature.
2. Full bath
3. Foot bath
4. Half bath
5. Pail douche. A shower may suffice. Pour water over the body of the patient who is sitting or standing in a bathtub. Swedish shampoo consists of brushing the body with a brush dipped in soapy water, using a circular motion on the skin to work up a lather. Pour a pail of water at 105° over the patient. Follow by a lukewarm shower. The Turkish shampoo is essentially the same, with the addition of a pail of water at 90° following the 105° pail pour.
6. Russian bath

7. Sponge bath
8. Vapor bath
9. Sitz bath, hot, neutral or cold
10. Shampoos—Use soap and water with fingertip massage in hairy areas.

Compresses

1. Heating compress: throat, chest, sinuses, skin lesions, boils, joints, chest wrapper and moist abdominal bandage
2. Hot or cold compresses or wet dressings with or without poultices of herbal extracts or teas
3. Wet girdle, moist abdominal bandage

Ice Applications

1. Ice water: applied by immersion of a part, by pouring through the hair or over the feet, and more commonly by compresses applied briefly
2. Block ice: applied by rubbing the part with a suitable size block of ice to achieve a vascular reaction or anesthesia

Irrigations

1. Enemas: hot, warm or cold; water, oil, or herbal tea
2. Nasal bath: applied with a bulb syringe or an electrical device such as a Water Pik
3. Vaginal douche: warm or hot; plain water, vinegar or baking soda, disinfectant, herbal tea as a styptic

Packs

1. Chest pack
2. Dripping sheet pack or wet sheet pack
3. Dry sheet pack
4. Fomentations
5. Half pack: same as wet sheet pack except that it is often used for patients who are too feeble to tolerate the full pack, and involves only part of the body
6. Leg pack
7. Shower pack: the wet sheet pack followed by frequent spraying from a hose or spray can, usually used as a refrigerant
8. Sweating pack: wet sheet pack covered with two or three thick blankets

Rubs and Friction

1. Rubbing wet sheet: dripping or wrung dry
2. Cold mitten friction, hot mitten friction, neutral mitten friction

3. Hand friction: dry rubbing or with hot or cold water (Friction can be controlled also by the use of talc, starch, alcohol or oil lubrication by simply varying the quantity of lubricant used)
4. Brush massage
5. Partial or full body rubs

Steam Applications

1. Tents
2. Towels
3. Specially designed chambers

Water Emetic, Lukewarm

The person should drink a glass or two of lukewarm water to induce vomiting.

Simple Equipment and Materials Needed

All equipment should be assembled and kept in a chest or box in ready access for instantaneous use. No search for materials or equipment should ever be required when the need arises.

Local Heat

Fomentation cloths
Tubs or bowls
Hot water bottles
Electric heat sources:
1. Heating pad or Thermophore
2. Electric light bulb (may use an inexpensive shop lamp)
3. Infrared bulb

Local Cold

Ice bag
Compress

Heating compress, moist abdominal bandage, wet girdle: various cloths, plastic and covers as described in the table below (Prepare these sets now and have them ready for use when needed. Pin the three parts together for storage, using a safety pin in one corner).

	Throat	Chest	Abdomen
Cotton cloth	2 × 14 × 20″	9 × 100″	10 × 50″
Plastic	3 × 14″	Plastic garbage bag	12 × 50″
Cover	4 × 34″	10 × 110″	12 × 55″

Poultices

Flaxseed
Hops or smartweed
Clay and glycerine
Comfrey
Charcoal

Tonic Friction

Basin and mitts for cold mitten friction
Sheet for sheet rubs

Sponging

Alcohol
Soap
Wash basin
Wash cloth

Rubs and Frictions

Oil
Massage lotion: half mineral oil, half alcohol, optional drop of oil of wintergreen for fragrance
Starch
Coarse salt for salt glow

Baths

Tub
Bathtub
Foot or arm tub
Sinus bowl
Electric light: custom built cabinet
Russian bath: custom built room

Packs

Whole blanket for full pack
Half or quarter blanket for hip or leg pack
Sheet for wet sheet packs

Spray and Douche

Shower equipped with needle spray
Pail for pour
Short hose 4-6 feet long for attachment to shower outlet, equipped with a nozzle to develop jets or sprays

Enema

Bag and nozzle
Bulb syringe
Oil
Herbals
Charcoal

Vaginal douche

Bag and nozzle
Vinegar
Baking soda
Disinfectant
Herbs for infection: garlic, charcoal, pekoe tea
Herbs as styptic: golden seal, witch hazel

DEFINITIONS OF WATER TEMPERATURE[78]

Possibly injurious	50° C.	Above 125° F. (even 110° in diabetes)
Painfully hot	42.8°-46° C.	110-120° F.
Very hot	40-42.8° C.	104-110° F.
Hot	38°-40° C.	100°-104° F.
Neutral	34.4° - 37° C.	94° - 97° F.
Warm	34° - 38° C.	92° - 100° F.
Tepid	27° - 34° C.	80° - 92° F.
Cool	21° - 27° C.	70° - 80° F.
Cold	13° - 21° C.	55° - 70° F.
Very Cold	0° - 13° C.	32° - 55° F.

Unfavorable Reactions in Hydrotherapy

1. Headache
   A. Placing feet in hot water actually causes rare individuals to get headaches, particularly if the water is very hot.
   B. The headache may also be caused by too long applications, excessive patient reaction, an incomplete reaction, or lack of sufficient reaction time in bed.
   C. Failure to accompany a heating treatment to the body with cold compresses to the head may cause headache. Any time the body temperature goes over 100° it is well to place a cool washcloth on the forehead and sponge the neck and face occasionally. This rule applies to fevers produced by disease as well as to the elevation in temperature caused by heating treatments.
2. Uncontrollable shivering
3. Vertigo
4. Insomnia
5. Palpitations
6. Extreme skin sensitivity with tickling, muscle guarding, or uncontrollable laughing
7. Hyperventilation syndrome
8. Faintness. Occasionally fainting is accompanied by muscle twitching or jerking.
9. Nausea

To correct an unpleasant reaction in hydrotherapy discontinue the treatment and wait 2-3 hours before attempting again. Immediately put the patient in a warm bath at 100° with or without friction to the back and extremities. Give one or two cups of catnip tea, cool or warm to meet the need. Coach the patient in a deep slow breathing exercise for 2-5 minutes. For palpitations, a gentle head-roll exercise will often be helpful, dropping the chin on the chest and making a tilt of the head first all around to the left, then all around to the right. Repeat only once or twice as the neck can get sore from overdoing it.

Misuse of Simple Remedies

Improperly Applied Remedies

Any simple remedy may be applied in a wrong fashion. Usually great knowledge or expertness are not required to understand that a remedy has been wrongly applied. An example is the overuse of sunlight in a fair-skinned individual.

Additionally, if a treatment is applied too hot or too cold, not hot enough or not cold enough, too short or too long a length of time, the patient may get an undesirable or uncomfortable reaction. If hydrotherapy is applied in a fashion judged to be not neat or appropriate by the patient, a failure to react may be mediated through the higher centers to the autonomic nervous system, then out to the precapillary sphincters controlling the circulation to result in a poor grade of reaction.

If the treatment fails to produce a vigorous surface circulation, the so-called incomplete reaction may occur. It is characterized by dusky or mottled skin, cutis anserina (gooseflesh), shivering, cold hands or feet, and a sense of fullness in the head, dizziness, nausea or faintness. The remedy for an incomplete reaction is often found in a hot foot bath. If the patient has a contraindication to a hot foot bath, such as hardening of the arteries of the lower extremities, use a hot compress to the lower abdomen and upper thighs to avoid injury.

It is more difficult to produce a good reaction in a person who has been drinking alcohol, and it is well to keep in mind that alcohol consumption does not warm the body. It does, however, increase the *sensation* of being warm at the same time that the skin is losing large quantities of heat from the surface. The core temperature can drop dangerously. The blood vessels react unreliably after alcohol consumption.

In order to be effective, some applications must be continued a certain minimum of time: a gargle should be at least ten minutes to be effective, and 20 minutes would be better. A two minute gargle will usually be ineffectual except to relieve discomfort temporarily.

Psychological or Nervous Factors

The patient may entertain certain mental attitudes which can interfere with a proper reaction. The effectiveness of the treatment depends on *both* the autonomic and the central nervous system. The autonomic nervous system is involved through its control over the precapillary sphincters, the production of releasing substances enabling the leukoyctes to be released from the bone marrow, and the manufacture of these and other proteins and antibodies to fight against disease. The central nervous system exerts a control over the treatment through the attitude of the patient, his nervousness, fear, critical attitude, even a lack of faith in the simple remedies; these can all be factors of a psychological or nervous nature which may interfere with a proper physiological reaction through the central nervous system. It is well-known that if a patient thinks the application of cold will make him get a sore throat, it is more likely to do so; if a patient thinks his food will hurt him, it more often does.

Heat Misused with Insulin

It is improper to apply heat to the extremities of an insulin-dependent diabetic. The diabetic more often than other patients has arterial disease with a reduction in the blood flow to an extremity. The application of heat increases the metabolism of the tissues, but does not increase the ability of the body to supply oxygen to the part. As a result, the metabolic needs can very quickly overuse the nutrients and oxygen available from the blood, and the cells can die from oxygen starvation on an acute basis simply through the application of heat. Therefore, hot foot baths are contraindicated in diabetes.

For any condition in a diabetic in which a hot foot bath is the treatment of choice, use instead a thick, large compress to the lower abdomen and upper thighs extending well along the sides, to get a reflex reaction in the lower extremities. In the young diabetic who has probably not developed arterial insufficiency, it is permissible to cautiously apply heat to the extremities. Diabetics also frequently develop a peripheral neuropathy making the involved parts (usually the feet) much less sensitive to all stimuli, in some cases being almost anesthetic. In such a situation, the patient cannot sense that the feet are getting too hot, and it would be very easy to burn the feet and cause severe damage.

Metabolism and Increased Temperature

It is improper to apply heat to the person or any body part if by so doing the increased metabolism or physiologic activity of the body or that part could cause injury. An example is the application of heat to a person with a failing heart or with a heart attack. In these cases it is desirable to keep the workload on the heart to a minimum. Therefore, it would be improper to cause the heart rate to rise significantly (over 20 beats per minute), through the application of total body heat. If it should be ascertained during any treatment that the cardiac reserve

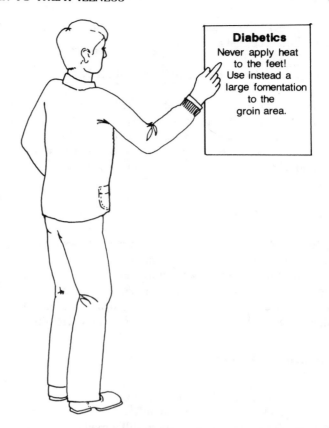

Diabetics
Never apply heat to the feet! Use instead a large fomentation to the groin area.

Insulin-dependent diabetics should not apply heat to the feet at a higher temperature than about 102° to 104°. The application should always be monitored carefully. Heating pads are dangerous for persons with poor arterial blood supply to the lower extremities as the amount of heat delivered to the skin cannot be accurately measured. A warm footbath can be tested by a thermometer, insuring a safe level. If there is any doubt, use a large fomentation to the groin to reflexively dilate the blood vessels in the feet.

is depleted, the treatment should be terminated and the pulse brought down through the application of a neutral bath or cool sponge.

Abscess May Be Prevented

Application of heat to an abscess in a closed space is often contraindicated. The application of heat to an infection tends to draw the infection to a central point, an undesirable occurence in a closed space. An example is that of the appendix. If acute appendicitis is caused to "collect" in the appendix, the appendix may swell and rupture. Similarly, an inflammation in a tooth should be scattered rather than collected into an abscess. Sometimes the application of heat in such cases, if an abscess pocket is already forming, will cause an increase in the patient's discomfort. If, however, the application of heat occurs early enough, the inflammation may subside and never reach the abscess stage.

Overtreatment and Undertreatment With Heat

Avoid overtreating the patient with too much heat, especially an unconscious patient, or an individual at the extremes of age, a child or an old person. Undertreatment is also possible, especially with the overuse of heat and the underuse of cold resulting in an "incomplete reaction."

Cold May be Misused

It is well to remember that some patients are hypersensitive to cold because of Raynaud's syndrome, which is the development of marked pallor or cyanosis of the extremities upon exposure to even mild cold, due to arterial spasm. Extremes of both heat and cold are contraindicated in marked arterial insufficiency of the extremities.

Treatment of Pain With Hydrotherapy

The application of heat or cold to relieve the pain of acute or chronic traumatic and inflammatory disorders has been used for centuries, and is still a method without peer in the area of pain control. No other method is so effective, so safe and easy, and so free from side effects and expense. Ice packs and other cold applications may be used in contusions and sprains during the first 24-48 hours. After the acute stage, either heat or cold may be used if pain continues.[85] Heat also may be properly used in acute injuries to control pain. If heat is used on contusions, sprains, and other acute injuries, however, it should be as hot as can be tolerated, usually above 110°, because of its greater ability to stop bleeding into the tissues above that temperature level. Very hot applications, above 110°, will stop capillary ooze into tissues as effectively as ice packs.

Cold packs will often relieve pain and reduce inflammatory edema in such disorders as sore throat, sinusitis, and appendicitis. In chronic conditions, heat is generally favored, though some patients find cold applications more effective and pleasant. In bursitis and arthritis most patients find that ice packs give greater relief of pain and stiffness, the average range of knee movement greatly improving after either heat or cold. However, in a bursa, or any closed space with fluid under tension, heat may increase the tension and aggravate the pain.

Cold water should be used to relieve the pain of burns. Immediately immerse the burned area in very cold or ice water or spray cold water over the area until the patient is free of pain. This treatment not only relieves pain, but reduces the extent of injury, inflammation and swelling, and often prevents blister formation. Cold water apparently reduces capillary permeability preventing subsequent swelling or blistering.

Heat or cold can often give some relief of headaches and other aches and pains of non-traumatic origin. Both are worth trying in persistent pain. Chronic low back pain will often be relieved by either ice packs or ice massage. Use a 4 to 8 ounce paper cup filled with water and frozen.

Wet bath towels can be refrigerated or placed in the freezer and then layered over a painful area. A proper size container of ice and water can be used for intermittent immersion of hand or foot. Wet or moist heat is generally more effective than dry heat, but many persons tolerate heating pads, steam packs, hydrocolators and Thermophore better than direct moist heat. Some patients like paraffin baths or paraffin gloves for relieving pain in arthritic hands better than other methods.

Referred Pain

The nerve impulses received from certain body parts enter the spinal cord at the same point as the nerve impulses from a diseased organ. This relationship may cause referred pain in the healthy part rather than in the diseased organ. When a painful stimulus arises in an area of low sensitivity which is in reflex connection with an area of high sensitivity, pain is felt in the area of high sensitivity. This phenomenon is known as allochiria.

Areas of Referred Pain[86] **Areas of Low Sensitivity**	**Reflex areas of High Sensitivity**
1. Heart and aorta	Dorsal segments 1, 2, 3, and 4
2. Lungs	Dorsal segments 1, 2, 3, 5, 6, and 7; most common 2 to 5.
3. Stomach	Dorsal segments 7-9
4. Intestines	Dorsal segments 9-11, and possibly 12
5. Liver, gallbladder	Dorsal segments 5-9
6. Kidney, ureter	Dorsal segment 10-12, Lumbar 1
7. Testis, ovary	Dorsal segment 10
8. Bladder	Sacral segments 3-4 for mucosa; pain of contraction in dorsal segments 11-12, and lumbar 1
9. Uterus, lower portion	Sacral segments 2-4
Upper portion	Dorsal 11-12, sometimes 10, and lumbar 1

Definitions in Hydrotherapy

1. Anodyne—an agent for the relief of pain
2. Antipyretic—an agent for lowering the body temperature
3. Antispasmodic—an agent for the relaxation of spasm or convulsion
4. Calorie—the same as specific heat, the standard of thermic measure: the amount of heat required to raise one gram of water one degree Celsius at 20° and sea level
5. Depletion—the result of derivation, the act of increasing the amount of blood in a part, reducing congestion
6. Depressant—similar to a sedative in which the various vital activities are decreased, but here more profoundly decreased, as seen in the reduction in basal metabolic rate with the prolonged chilling of the thyroid
7. Derivative—a measure for drawing blood or lymph from a particular part by increasing the blood or lymph in another part
8. Diaphoresis—the act of producing sweating
9. Diuresis—the act of increasing the production of urine
10. Eliminative—a procedure which promotes the excretion of urine, sweat, breath, or feces
11. Excitant—that which increases the activity or output
12. Fluxion—the act of greatly increasing the circulation to a single part, such as to the spinal cord or to an extremity, renewing the blood supply and washing out accumulated toxins
13. Inflammation—a condition in which there are redness, heat, swelling and pain, the four cardinal signs of inflammation. There are several processes combined to produce inflammation; it may be caused by an infection such as by germs and their toxins or by bruising, chemical irritation, or strain of the part as in overworked muscles. I believe that inflammation tends to be scattered by both cold and heat when applied early in the course of an abscess, but heat tends to collect the inflammation into a pus pocket when applied later on. If the body resources are so stimulated that the inflammation is reduced or scattered without collecting pus into an abscess there will be less tissue destruction. Pus is formed from dead tissue products, edema fluid, white blood cells, and sometimes germs. Any time pus collects it is best to drain the pus from the tissues to promote quick healing. If the pus is not drained, it will need to be reabsorbed into the circulation, a slow process.
14. Latent heat—the amount of heat in terms of calories necessary to convert a material from one state to another without changing its temperature (Example: ice changes to water by storing 80 calories per gram of water. Water changes to steam by storing 540 calories per gram of water. The calories thus stored are given off when the change is made back to the previous form of water, e.g., in the change from steam to condensed water).
15. Lumen—the interior of any tubular structure
16. Refrigerant—an agent for cooling the body, usually at the same time relieving thirst and restoring the alkalinity of the blood, such as by free water drinking
17. Revulsive—usually pertains to the application of heat followed by a brief application of cold
18. Sedative—an agent which decreases the vital activities to below par. It is usually conducive to relaxation and sleep
19. Specific Heat—the amount of heat required to raise one gram of water one degree Celsius from 20° C. to 21° C. at sea level
20. Spoliative—a treatment to increase the oxidation, or the catabolic action of a tissue. The usual intended function is to reduce weight.
21. Stimulant—increases vital activities above par. The body is aroused to unusual activities. The vital activities are increased, but to a higher degree than usual, either above the present or above the normal function of that particular tissue or organ. There are various degrees such as mild, moderate, and marked.
22. Sudoresis—same as diaphoresis
23. Tonic—an agent to restore body activities to par. The effect of increasing vital activities so as to restore the body to normal tone or to increase the tone of the body above the normal. The nutrition, circulation, and other body functions are promoted.
24. Vasodilatation—the act of increasing the diameter of blood vessels or lymph vessels
25. Vasomotor—pertaining to the motion of the blood vessels

CHAPTER ELEVEN

Techniques

1. FULL FOMENTATIONS WITH ALTERNATING HOT AND COLD (REVULSIVE)

Fomentation Pack (Steam Pack) and Cover
A. Steam pack of one of the following materials:

1. 50% synthetic or wool, with 50% cotton
2. Brushed cotton canvas type
3. Other loosely woven but substantial blanket material
4. Thick terry cloth or Turkish towels cut or folded to make about 4 thicknesses

Wool has a drawback in that it gives off an unpleasant odor on heating, but holds heat nicely. The piece of material for the first three types above should be 36″ × 30″ or 31″ and should be folded in thirds so that the finished dimensions are approximately 12″ × 31″. For terry cloth or Turkish towels, cut or fold the material so that the finished product will be four thicknesses, and measuring 12″ × 30″. Sew the pack together at both ends, or make about 6 quilting stitches with heavy thread tied securely, to hold the ends in place. Different size packs may be made by varying either length or width. Cravat packs can be made by doubling a piece of material 8″ × 14″ to 4″ × 14″, which will fit the adult neck.

B. The pack cover should be a wool or acrylic piece measuring 34″ × 34″ for general use, or correspondingly altered in size for special areas. Fomentation covers must be large enough to overlap all parts of the pack and could be as large as 40″ × 32″ to 36″. They may be made of synthetic blanket material, a light-weight, easily laundered, moisture resistant material. Neither the pack nor the cover should be of stiff material as the pack should drape easily around the body contours.

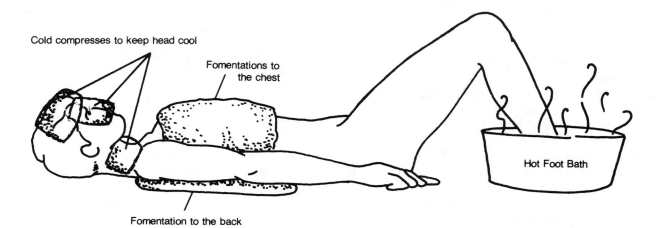

Cold compresses to keep head cool

Fomentations to the chest

Fomentation to the back

Hot Foot Bath

Full fomentations include a steam pack to the back, a series of three steam packs to the chest, a hot foot bath kept quite warm, and cold compresses to the face, head, or neck. The steam pack at the back may extend the full length of the spine, from the neck to the coccyx for the maximum reaction.

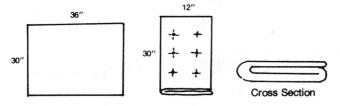

Cross Section

The fomentation pack is made easily from many types of material. Here shown is a 30 x 36" piece of thick, brushed cotton laundry flannel folded in thirds and fastened by quilting with thread, string, or colored yarn.

Equipment for Fomentation.

1. Three or four fomentation packs as hot as can be tolerated
2. Two to four fomentation covers
3. Four Turkish towels
4. Two wash cloths, for cold compresses, and cold mitten friction
5. One or two patient sheets (Extra sheet and blanket may be needed).
6. One foot tub with water approximately 105° to 110°
7. One basin with cold or ice water
8. One glass and straw
9. A canner or other large kettle rigged with a false bottom or rack

Procedure

1. If uncertain, consult chart for reflex areas to determine best location for application of treatment.
2. Protect the bed by a doubled blanket or a plastic sheet such as shower curtain.
3. Assist the patient to undress and drape in sheet.
4. Place one or two fomentations for the spine on the bed and cover well with towels to prevent burning the patient.
5. Assist the patient to lie on the fomentation and place feet in a hot foot bath, if the area to be treated is such that the patient can lie in a supine position. If another position is to be used, wrap the feet well in a fomentation or surround them with hot water bottles.
6. Arrange necessary towels (1-4 thicknesses) over the area to be treated.
7. Place the fomentation neatly in position and cover it with a towel, sheet, and blanket if necessary.
8. Remove the fomentation after the desired length of time, usually 3-6 minutes, and replace it promptly with a cold compress for 30-60 seconds; dry the skin after the cold application.

9. Use a cold compress to the head or throat after 3-5 minutes, or when sweating begins.
10. Have the patient drink water, room temperature or hotter.
11. Inquire as to tolerance; perhaps more hot water could be added to the foot tub. The skin may get too hot at sensitive points.
12. Repeat numbers 6, 7 and 8 two or three times or more depending on the case, spending as little time during changes as possible.
13. Rub the thighs with a dry towel to remove perspiration.
14. Keep the foot bath hot by frequent additions of hot water, using care to avoid discomfort (see special instructions for a hot foot bath).
15. If indicated, give a cold mitten friction, soothing back rub, or shower to finish. Otherwise pat or rub briskly to dry or give an alcohol rub. Allow no wasted time as it is important to finish promptly to allow the reaction to proceed unhindered. There should be no hint of haste, but a calm, unhurried (never dawdling) demeanor should be manifested by all in the treatment room.
16. Before removing the hot foot tub, pour cold water over the feet and dry well between the toes.

Reflex Areas

Apply treatment to hatched areas

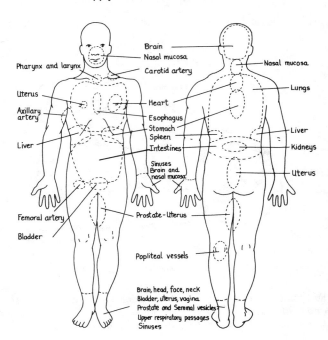

Precautions

1. Avoid drafts, noise, interruptions.
2. Avoid chilling and unnecessary fanning.
3. Avoid burning with hot fomentations.
4. Expose only the part under treatment.
5. Observe patient carefully for comfort, safety, and proper reaction.

Effects

1. Pain relief when used very hot for 3 to 5 minutes. Omit the cold compress in pleurisy, dysmenorrhea, and in arthritis if pain worsens when cold is applied.
2. Flushing and cleansing of tissues
3. Mobilizing white blood cells to fight infection
4. A tonic in apathetic states if the fomentations are brief and very hot
5. A stimulus to blood circulation when brief, very hot applications are followed by short, very cold compresses
6. Soothing for the nerves if moderate and prolonged— 6-10 minutes—for spasm of muscles or tension
7. Sweat production to increase toxin elimination

Contraindications

1. Diabetes—do not apply to the feet.
2. Paralyzed or unconscious patients—do not use due to danger of burning.
3. Heart attacks—take care to place an ice bag over the heart before fomentations are laid on.

A treatment given tenderly and with sympathy and tact will do more good than the most skilled treatment given in a cold, indifferent way. "Why need anyone be ignorant of God's remedies—hot-water fomentations and cold and hot compresses."[87] The prayer of thanksgiving should be constantly in the heart for the goodness, forethought, and wisdom of our Heavenly Father for the simple remedies which are so effective, comforting, and readily available to all.

Keep the Head Cool

Ice bags placed on the forehead lower the temperature of the brain by 1.5° although the cold applied to the skin of the forehead does not cause chilling of the tissue deeper than about 1 cm. There are reflex reactions between the skin and the deeper structures which alter the blood flow within the deep organs immediately beneath the skin surface when heat, cold, or irritants are applied to the surface. These are called cutaneo-visceral reflexes. It is by means of these reflexes that the brain temperature is lowered when cold compresses are applied to the forehead.

There is a depression of electroencephalographic (EEG) activity as the body temperature goes above 104°. While abnormal waves have been observed in some studies on patients with far-advanced cancer, there appears to be the likelihood that the widespread disease, possibly cerebral metastasis, could have been the aggravating factor in those cases, and not the elevation of temperature. In febrile convulsions in children it appears that the toxic element producing the fever is the stimulating source for the convulsions and not the increased temperature, an agent that in itself causes an actual depression of EEG activity.[88]

Cold applications to the head are used to prevent congestion of the brain, or to relieve congestion if it is already present. The application of cold to the head is usually in the form of a cold towel compress; but an ice cap, an ice collar, or a poultice of ice are sometimes used for special purposes. Cold sponging of the face is also advantageous. The effort to keep the head cool may include cold compresses to the neck, if the heat applied to the body is very intense, or very prolonged. Generally speaking, all hot and warm applications and many local applications such as the hot foot bath should be accompanied by cool or cold to the head, particularly if the treatment lasts longer than about seven minutes, or if the body temperature is expected to rise higher than 100°.

In some individuals, the application of heat to a localized area of the body results in dilatation of the blood vessels of the brain, making it desirable to apply cold to the head to prevent congestion. The application of cold causes contraction of the carotid and vertebral arteries in all their branches.[89]

In this way the amount of blood which flows to the brain is decreased and the temperature of the brain is reduced. Even sitz baths and wet sheet packs should be accompanied by cold compresses to the face and head when the patient begins to heat up.

2. FEVER TREATMENTS, INSTITUTIONAL USE

In many cases, a temperature of 106° can be obtained in 60 to 70 minutes. In other patients, 90 minutes will be required before the temperature reaches this level. Rectal readings are taken every 10 or 15 minutes. At 106°, the patient may lose from two to five pounds of water and develop considerable weakness and discomfort because of dehydration. There may be a loss of one-third of the body stores of chloride. The patient should be made to drink from one to four quarts of 0.6% solution of sodium chloride during a five hour session. To make the solution, put two level teaspoons of table salt in each quart of water.[90]

In some patients the pulse increases to 120 and holds for the remainder of the treatment, but in some it may reach to 140 and 150. The patient must be closely watched for signs of exhaustion. If the pulse rises toward 160, it should be regarded as a danger signal and the temperature immediately reduced about one-half degree, or whatever is necessary to bring pulse down to 140 or below. The systolic blood pressure may increase 20 to 30 points during the first hour, then fall gradually to 10 to 50 points below the initial pressure. The diastolic pressure usually remains steady or falls slightly. If the pulse pressure, the difference between systolic and diastolic readings, falls to 20, terminate the treatment and consider this a sign of cardiovascular insufficiency. Simply give a neutral bath or a cool sponge and the pulse should return promptly to the pre-treatment level in a few minutes. Be sure to have fresh, cool, dry air in the treatment room for patients with a low cardiac reserve. Even more care than ordinary should be used to keep the head cool in these patients, and a physician should be constantly present in the treatment area when fevers over 105° are being administered.

A few patients become slightly delirious or dreamy during the fever treatment, probably because of drifting into a light level of sleep; they may talk in the sleep. Most patients get at least one period of drowsiness. Others may get a degree of excitement, agitation, inability to express thoughts, faintness or nervousness. The absence of toxicity in artificial fevers makes the patient more comfortable during the treatment than during a natural fever of the same degree. The more determined the person is to get well, the better the self-control, and the fewer unpleasant symptoms expressed. The patient must not be left alone until the session has been completed and the temperature returns to normal. Fever treatments in older patients with oral temperatures above 105° are a fairly strenuous test of cardiovascular function and must be supervised carefully. Tuberculosis is a contraindication to fever therapy because of diminished respiratory efficiency.

In contrast to other modalities of treatment, artificial fever produces no chills, shock, or toxic reactions to work against the body's defense mechanisms. The peak increase in neutrophilic white blood cells occurs an hour or two after the cessation of artificial fever, and lymphocytes begin to increase several hours later, even up to 24 hours and continue elevated for several days. Respirations increase by five to six per minute per degree of increase in temperature. It is believed that hot baths, even brief, stimulate the body's immune mechanism and treat the cause of the fever, not just the elevation in core temperature.

Therapeutic Complications of Fever Treatments

About 45% of patients receiving fever treatments over 105° orally will complain of headache which lasts a few hours. About 30% of patients will have some nausea and vomiting. An occasional patient with temperature over 105° will have tetany, muscular pain, muscular fibrillation, fainting, loss of consciousness, mild delirium, small blisters on the skin, and fever blisters or labial herpes (about 10%). In one hospital in the thirties, of 362 patients treated with artificial fever up to 107°, one death was reported in a young woman, previously healthy, who, nearing the end of the first session of treatment suddenly collapsed while still in the treatment room and died immediately. The factor or factors responsible for her death were not determined.[85] There have been no deaths reported at oral temperatures below 105°. We recommend that the higher temperatures be used only for certain special disorders and then only when the direct supervision of a physician is continuously available. Fevers up to 102° are safe and comfortable in a home situation and may be easily self-administered.

It should be remembered that red blood cells may have an increased fragility with even small increases in body temperature. Fever treatment can be used to advantage to treat elevated blood counts, but may not be as beneficial to treat anemia. Frequent hematocrits should be obtained in anemic patients receiving fever treatments.[86]

Indications for Fever Treatments

1. Colds (100° to 103°)
2. Influenza (100° to 103°)
3. Pain anywhere in the body (100° to 103°)
4. High blood pressure (101°)
5. Sore throat or quinsy (100° to 103°)
6. Viral infections such as Herpes, shingles, etc. (102° to 103°)
7. Lupus or rheumatoid diseases (100° to 103°)
8. Gonorrhea (106° to 107°)
9. Syphilis (106° to 107°)
10. Other venereal diseases (104° to 107°)
11. Arthritis (101° to 103°)
12. Cancer (102° to 104°)
13. Impetigo (102°)
14. Multiple sclerosis: never self-administered, as some patients get weak (100° to 104°)
15. Nephritis or kidney failure (100° to 101°)
16. Many other diseases (The severity and nature determine the degree of fever).

Contraindications to Fever Treatments

1. Low blood pressure (may cause fainting)
2. Heart diseases
3. Toxic thyroid
4. Alkalotic states of metabolism. Fever treatments themselves produce alkalosis because of hyperventilation. There is, however, no increase in the potassium concentration in artificial fevers.[94]
5. Tuberculosis
6. Blood loss or anemia

Equipment for Fever Treatments

1. Basin of ice water
2. 2-4 washcloths
3. 2-4 towels
4. Oral thermometer
5. Bath thermometer
6. Small electric fan for the face (optional)
7. Cushion or pillow for head
8. Stool or chair for attendant
9. Glass and straw for water

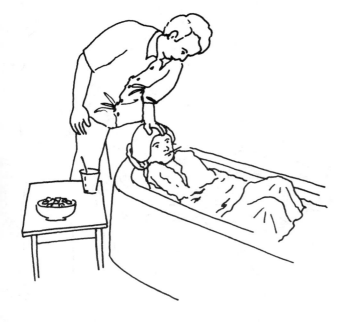

Fever treatment in a bathtub—Keep a thermometer in the patient's mouth. The temperature may go up to 102° or 103°. Give water generously by mouth. Use two towels to cover the patient, one for the knees, and one for the shoulders. A folded towel or plastic cushion may be used as a pillow for the head.

Procedure for the Russian Bath as a Fever Treatment

Fever treatments may be administered in a number of ways: whirlpool bath, electric light box, Russian steam cabinet, blanket pack, and bathtub. Frequent fever treatments are weakening because of mineral losses and should not be taken more than 5 times weekly, less frequently in weak or very sick patients.

A room about 8′ × 4.5′ × 6.5′ should be provided with a door on the right and a small window on the left at the level of the bed for the patient's head to project through. A cot should be provided that abuts against the wall immediately beneath the window. Have a 4″ foam pad covered with plastic. A headrest which is built onto the outside of the window should be fashioned with a similar 4″ foam pad and a pillow for the patient's head. A spiral screen door spring can be strung across the top of the window for a towel rack to provide privacy for the patient. The window should be approximately 1½′ square.

During the treatment the patient is placed on the table which has been prepared by a sheet over the plastic pad cover, and a hot fomentation for the patient to lie upon. A hot foot bath may be provided for the patient, or the patient's feet may be allowed to be exposed to the steam. The patient's head projects through the window and the therapist sits beside the patient's head with a bowl of ice water and a small electric fan for the face. The steam is turned on in the room and the air temperature adjusted at about 130° to 135°. The patient's oral temperature will rise to 102° in about 10 to 30 minutes. At that time the temperature in the room should be reduced to about 110° until the patient's temperature rises to 104°. At this time the room temperature is further reduced to 108° or 106°, and kept at just the proper temperature to maintain the patient's temperature at 104° to 105° for one-half to five hours, depending on the illness being treated. The pulse should not be allowed to rise above 160 under any circumstance, and generally the pulse should stabilize at about 120 to 130.

Give the patient copious quantities of water or saline, generally administered hot. The patient's face should be frequently sponged with a cold compress, about every two minutes, and more frequently in fevers above 104°.

The Electric Light Bath

Definition

A specially-designed cabinet with a floor space 5 feet square and about 4½ feet tall holds 80 bare-filament incandescent lights of about 60-100 watts arranged in four

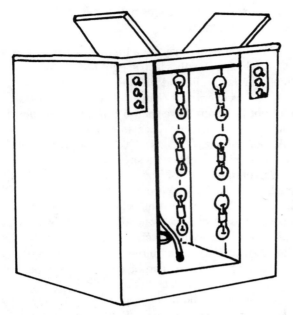

The electric light cabinet is useful for institutional work. It can be built inexpensively for home use. Put about 20 bulbs in each of the four corners of the cabinet, 80 in all. Use 6 switches and two circuits, as all 80 bulbs on one outlet can overload the circuit. The patient sits in the cabinet, head projecting from the top and a heavy curtain hung for a door.

strips, one in each corner. The patient enters the cabinet from the side, that side having been left without a wall. A heavy sheet, blanket or canvas is hung over the open side. A fold-in shutter arrangement with a hole cut in the top is made so that the head projects from the hole in the top, the excess space being covered by a towel draped around the patient's neck. The patient sits in the cabinet, head projecting from the box, side and top sealed off by the canvas sheet and the neck towel. It is best if the 4 strips of light bulbs are designed for a separate switch to operate one third of the lights, 6 switches being required to turn on all lights. To prevent circuit overload, put half the bulbs on one circuit to plug in one outlet, and the other half on another.

The beginning air temperature in the cabinet is around 70°, but in a few minutes reaches 125° or 130°. The body temperature rises nicely to 101° to 102° in about 20 minutes. Sweating begins in 5-8 minutes and should be the signal to start the facial sponging to keep the head cool. A cold cloth laid over the bridge of the nose, cheeks, eyes, and forehead, molded to the facial structures will feel very comforting.

Remove the patient when the desired temperature is reached, or after 10-20 minutes in the bath. Finish with a cold mitten friction, a cool shower, or a full body massage.

Indications

For any acute or chronic condition requiring fever treatment, the electric light bath may prove the most comfortable mode of administration. If the person has a fever due to toxins or some subacute or acute inflammatory condition, there is usually a sharp fall of 1° to 2°, many times occurring 10-15 minutes after the bath. Colds and flu are nicely treated with the electric light bath.

Any condition making sweating desirable can be treated well by the electric light bath. It is helpful as a sedative and sudorific for drug withdrawal, tobacco cessation, and alcohol withdrawal. It is useful in agitated, anxious or depressed states.[97]

3. HOT FOOT BATH WITH BLANKET PACK (HOT MUSTARD IMMERSION BATH)

The hot foot bath is one of the most useful of all hydrotherapeutic measures. Perhaps if we had only one hydrotherapeutic measure available to us, we would need to select the hot foot bath. It has so many uses, so few contraindications, and is so readily available under all kinds of forbidding circumstances. It requires only inexpensive equipment and other expendable items.

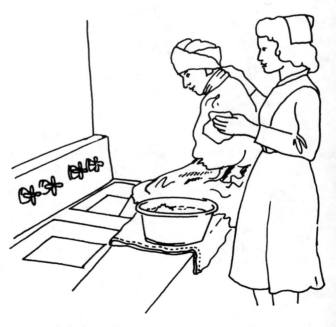

The hot footbath. A child may sit on the side of a sink or the kitchen deck for a hot footbath. An adult can put a small tub or large pan under the spigot while sitting on the edge of the bathtub. In this way the water can be kept hot easily from the nearby spigot.

General Instructions

1. The patient may be prepared in a number of ways, including lying in bed, the footbath to be placed in the bed on a towel or plastic sheet to protect the bed.
2. The patient may be seated fully dressed on the side of a bathtub, a smaller foot tub being used inside the bathtub, under the spigot to easily replenish the hot water. With a simple foot bath for the relief of early symptoms of a cold or sore throat, or the restoration of normal body temperature after chilling, the patient may be dressed in ordinary clothes; no further preparation than the removal of the foot gear need be done, and the body temperature need not be elevated significantly above normal.
3. The patient may be seated in a chair with a blanket wrap to be used during the foot bath. If the treatment is expected to result in sweating and an elevation of the body temperature by several degrees, the patient should be undressed and wrapped in a sheet, several blankets being used to retain the body heat, and the sheet being used to absorb the sweat.

Equipment

1. Foot tub or large basin (in a pinch use a trash can) about half filled with hot water (100° to 110°) preferably to 3-8 inches above the ankles
2. Pitcher of very hot water
3. Sheets or treatment blankets, according to the climate and patient's condition
4. One or two Turkish towels
5. Wash cloths for head compress
6. Basin of ice water
7. Bath thermometer useful
8. Dry mustard (1 teaspoon per gallon of water) or powdered horseradish or other irritant if desired

Procedure

1. Drape one or two blankets to completely cover a straight chair, and cover the blanket entirely with a sheet.
2. Place a Turkish towel on the floor for protection with a tub of hot water on it. Put the dry mustard in the water if maximal redness of the skin is desirable, as in headache.
3. Seat the undressed patient on the chair with the feet in the tub, and wrap snugly, first in the sheet and then in the blankets, draping covers well about the tub and patient's knees to avoid the circulation of air. A towel can be wrapped around the neck to hold the

blankets snugly in place, and to catch the sweat from the face and head.
4. Apply cold compress to forehead. Change every 2-3 minutes during the height of the reaction.
5. Add hot water frequently during the treatment to keep the temperature up to the patient's tolerance.
6. Continue treatment for 20 to 30 minutes or even an hour or more if needed. Give water to drink when sweating begins.
7. To terminate treatment hold feet up with one hand and dash or pour cold water over them. Be sure to cover both dorsal and plantar surface.
8. Place the feet on a towel on the floor. Avoid even a one-second contact with the chilled floor as an entirely different reaction may occur than from the cold water pour.
9. Dry the skin thoroughly, especially between the toes.
10. Have the patient lie down for 30 to 60 minutes for the reaction time.

Effects

1. Relieves headaches, congestion in eyes, earaches, dysmenorrhea; useful for pelvic and prostatic conditions, sore throat, gallstone, renal colic, and many other disorders
2. Decreases internal congestion anywhere
3. Aids in sweating (nephritis, toxic states)
4. Prepares for a cold treatment
5. Relaxes and reduces fatigue
6. Prevents or shortens a cold or influenza
7. Warms a chilled person
8. Relieves abdominal pain
9. Substitutes for a hot half bath in pregnant woman and others who should not be given fever treatments or total body heating treatments

Precautions

1. In adding hot water to the foot bath, push the feet to one side, and place your hand between the feet and the hot water. Pour the hot water against the tub and swirl it with your hand.
2. If the patient perspires, dry the limbs thoroughly. The thighs are especially likely to perspire.
3. Do not end with cold preceding a massage of the feet or during menstruation.

Contraindications

1. Diabetes, insulin-dependent
2. Buerger's disease

3. Arteriosclerosis of lower extremities
4. Loss of feeling in feet or legs
5. Unconsciousness

4. COLD FOOT BATH

Indications

1. Any condition requiring reflex contraction of the blood vessels of the brain, pelvic organs and bladder, liver or gastrointestinal tract
2. Uterine bleeding, post-partum hemorrhage
3. Bladder or kidney bleeding

Contraindications

1. Chilled patient
2. Extreme fear of chilling
3. Active menstruation, unless used to check heavy flow
4. During a headache except migraine
5. Acute pulmonary inflammations
6. Asthma

Procedure

1. Put water in the foot tub to about 2-4 inches depth at 40° to 60°.
2. Treatment time is 20 to 150 seconds for contraction of blood vessels.
3. Longer treatment times may cause reflex dilatation of blood vessels in the same areas.
4. The feet may be rubbed or brushed during the treatment if desired.
5. Dry the feet thoroughly.
6. Post-treatment reaction time is 45 to 60 minutes in bed.

5. FLUXION TO SPINE

Fluxion is a quickening of the rate at which blood passes through a part. The effect is achieved in one of three ways: (1) by an increase in the pressure on the arterial tree, (2) by opening up the arteries so that they carry a larger volume of blood, (3) by increasing the pressure on the venous side of the circulation. The blood is the great healer. It washes out wastes and toxins, and brings in fresh elements to heal the diseased tissues. Increased movement of blood and lymph is therefore primary to any healing process.

The superficial blood vessels in most parts of the body act reciprocally. As an illustration of this principle,

let us suppose we apply a cold compress over a fleshy part, such as the front of the thigh. A resulting reduction in flow of blood to the skin will be accompanied by an increase in blood to the underlying quadriceps femoris muscle. If, on the other hand, a hot fomentation is applied to the skin, the result will be a diversion of blood to the skin and relatively less to the underlying muscle.

In states of congestion of the brain or spinal cord, the application of alternating hot and cold from the back of the head to the tip of the spine acts as a vigorous stimulant and tonic measure. It is given in the same manner as the full fomentation with revulsion, the fomentation being laid on the back for 3-4 minutes, and instead of the cold compress, a small piece of ice is quickly rubbed up and down five to ten times. The back is then dried and another fomentation applied. The next fomentation should be ready before the ice is used.

This treatment reduces congestion and improves the circulation and vasomotor tone in the spinal cord and brain.

6. THE DRY BLANKET PACK

This treatment is the same as described in the hot foot bath with blanket pack, merely omitting the hot foot bath. A hot water bottle may be placed under the feet, and also against the flanks. This treatment is for the purpose of warming up a patient, but a slight fever can be obtained if it is prolonged.

7. KIDNEY STONE PACK

Very large, very hot fomentations are needed and should be applied quickly, while the heat is still almost unbearable. Maintain the hot application and keep it hot with a hot water bottle or electric device for maintaining heat. Keep the head cool by cold compresses.

For a kidney stone treatment, spread a half-sheet across the middle of the bed. On it place a heating pad turned up to high, with a sturdy plastic square or garbage bag to cover it; over this place a hot pack and then a towel. Position the patient with the kidney area (slightly above the waist) centered over this pack. Bring up the sheet on each side and pin it snugly around the body so as to hold the pack in place. Keep it hot for hours with the heating pad if necessary, until the stone passes or the patient gets relief from pain. Plug a radio into the same electrical outlet with the heating pad. In the event moisture accidently gets on the electric units, the short will cause static on the radio. The volume of the radio should be turned on loudly enough to be heard easily, and then the radio tuned to a silent area on the dial.

8. THE COLD COMPRESS

A cloth wrung from cold water or salt water (NaCl, epsom salt, boric acid) or herbal steep may be applied to any body surface.

Equipment

1. Cloths or cotton fabric pieces. Wash cloths are convenient.
2. Cold or ice water, or desired solution

Procedure

1. Wring the cloth from cold water; it should be dry enough so it won't drip and yet wet enough to stay cold for awhile. Lay it on the skin, molding it around body parts and folding it to fit the area.
2. Avoid wetting the hair when treating the head, face, or throat.
3. Renew frequently. Sometimes, when adequate protection is used, a few ice chips may be placed in the folds of the cloth.
4. Occasionally wipe the whole area with a cold cloth.
5. Dry thoroughly at conclusion.

Effects and Uses

1. Produces a comfortable sensation when used on the face, forehead or neck of a patient who is being heated and sweating freely
2. Narrowing of the blood vessels with a decrease in local blood flow and a marked decrease in local congestion
3. Decreases pain, itching, and swelling; ideal for some rashes, for drying of weeping areas, and for loosening scales
4. Reduces fever when applied to over one-fourth of the body
5. Slows heart, increases force of heartbeat, and raises blood pressure
6. Medicated compresses for special purposes: antibacterial, antifungal, and anti-inflammatory. Garlic water may be used, as may comfrey, golden seal, mint, or potato water.
7. Additional uses listed under wet dressings

Contraindications

1. Do not use in a chilled patient.
2. Do not use for pleurisy or sinusitis as symptoms may worsen.

9. ICE PACK OR ICE BAG

Indications

1. Sprains, strains
2. Tennis elbow
3. Backache
4. Appendicitis or salpingitis
5. Toothache
6. Headache
7. In heating treatments, used for the head when oral temperature is over 101°
8. Pain
9. Bursitis
10. Goiter
11. Swelling
12. Bleeding
13. Congestion
14. Inflammation
15. Rapid or weak heart action

Contraindications

1. Worsening of symptoms with use
2. Extreme aversion to cold
3. Headache or Raynaud's symptoms upon contact with cold

Precaution

To avoid injury of the tissues be certain that the tissues are not in direct contact with the ice.

Procedure for Several Methods

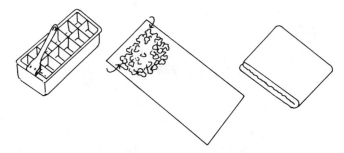

1. Put one tray of ice cubes in a small face towel. Fold it over to make a loose pack about 5″ x 10″. This is very easily used on the top of the head, the back of the neck, or the right lower abdominal quadrant.
2. Put one tray of ice cubes in a plastic bread bag or similar plastic bag. Arrange the pieces of ice loosely so that a flat pack about 5″ x 10″ will be produced.

Lay it on a pillow and place the heel in the middle of the pack to treat a sprain. A second pack may be needed to lay over the ankle. Cover with a towel. Leave in place for 20 minutes for a sprain, 5-10 minutes for tennis elbow or bursitis.

3. Commercial ice bags in various sizes and shapes are suitable for use on the head, foot or spine (3 x 10″). Fill the bag or icecap about half full with finely chopped ice. Dry the surface and cover with a hand towel.

4. Ice cravats can be made easily by placing ice on a towel and folding in such a way that the cravat is about 3 inches wide and long enough to encircle the neck. A commercial plastic collar can be filled with crushed ice in the same manner as the icecap. Ice collars or cravats are useful in fevers, congestive headache, meningitis, sunstroke, and when prolonged sweating treatments are given, as in eclampsia or kidney failure.

10. ALTERNATE HOT AND COLD IMMERSION BATHS

A body part may be immersed alternately in hot and cold water.

Equipment

1. Two containers (garbage pails, foot tubs, baby bathtubs, five gallon cans, etc.) large enough to allow water to generously cover the areas to be treated along with the adjacent parts
2. Bath thermometer
3. Towels
4. Sheets

Procedure

1. Place the part in hot water (105° to 110°) for three to four minutes. If a finger is to be treated, the whole hand and wrist should be immersed. If the ankle is to be treated, immerse the foot and leg up to mid-calf.
2. Now place the part in cold water, tap or ice, for 30 to 60 seconds.
3. While the part is in cold water, add hot water to increase the temperature of the hot bath or at least to maintain the temperature. Do not exceed 120°, even in a vigorous young person; usually milder temperatures are adequate to give the maximum reaction possible, and a more intense application cannot produce a greater reaction.
4. Begin the treatment in the hot and end in the cold.

5. Make six to eight complete changes, unless the treatment is being given to reduce swelling in which case the treatment should continue until the swelling begins to go down, perhaps an hour or two.
6. Dry thoroughly, handling carefully such injuries as sprains.

Effects

1. Reduces pain, locally and in a distant part
2. May alternate contraction and dilatation of blood vessels, or enhance dilatation
3. Markedly increases blood flow
4. Increases white blood cells in the circulation, both the number of cells and their activity
5. Increases local metabolic effects
6. Increases phagocytic and immunity responses
7. Reduces swelling

Precautions

1. Use a cold compress to head if there is a tendency to sweat during the treatment.
2. Cool the patient during the post-treatment reaction by putting the patient to bed for about 30 minutes.
3. Hot water must not be over 103° in peripheral vascular disease of the lower extremities as is often the case in advanced, insulin-dependent diabetes.
4. A disinfectant such as lysol may be used in the water. Clean the equipment thoroughly when an open or infected wound is present.

11. STEAM BATH OR CHAIR SWEAT

Equipment

1. A simple straight chair
2. Pot or kettle filled with water
3. Hotplate
4. Sheet, blanket, or fire-proof plastic cover
5. Three towels, one for draping around neck, one to turban the hair, and one for the seat
6. Ice bag
7. Wrist watch or clock with a second hand
8. Glass of hot water for drinking
9. Hot foot bath equipment
10. Oil of eucalyptus or mint if medicated steam is needed, about 1 teaspoon of oil or 2 tablespoons of dried mint leaves per pot of water

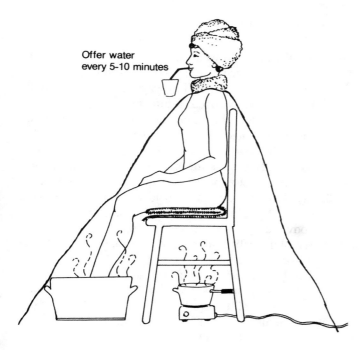

Offer water every 5-10 minutes

Procedure

1. Place hot plate and pot of boiling water under the chair seat. Fold a towel and place it in the seat of chair. Put a tub of hot water in place for the hot foot bath.
2. Seat the undressed, turbaned patient on the towel and begin the hot foot bath. When sweating begins or oral temperature exceeds 100°, apply the cold compresses to the head. Keep the foot bath hot by adding hot water.
3. Drape the sheet or blanket or both, or the fire-proof plastic cover in tent fashion around the back and shoulders to cover the body from the neck down, including the foot bath, so that the steam from the boiling pot is captured. Use care if a tea kettle is used that the spout is not directed toward the patient.
4. Fold a towel lengthwise and fashion as a snug-fitting collar to hold the sheet in place and prevent steam from escaping.
5. Encourage the patient to drink one to two glasses of hot water to encourage sweating.
6. Check mouth temperature and pulse at temple or neck. Keep the pulse under 140 and the oral temperature under 104°. Keep the air temperature under the tent between 120° and 130° until the body temperature goes up to 102°-104°, when it can be reduced to 105°-110°.
7. After removing the steam apparatus and drying the feet, the sweating and fever can be prolonged by

blankets, the patient going from chair to bed still wrapped in the tent sheet. Cover warmly with blankets to prolong the sweating. The treatment may be terminated with a shower or cold mitten friction as desired.
8. Give one-half to one hour of reaction time in bed. If sweating has been profuse, have the patient take a cleansing shower at the end of the reaction time to cleanse the skin and readjust skin temperature. Administer copious amounts of water by mouth during and after the treatment.

Precautions

1. The patient should be vigorous and basically healthy, not debilitated or feeble.
2. Keep a constant watch over the patient, checking vital signs frequently. Take pulse and temperature readings every 15 minutes until temperature is above 103°, then every 5 minutes until the temperature is again below 103°.

Effects

1. Produces profuse sweating
2. Opens up sinuses
3. Increases metabolism
4. Fights a cold, influenza, or "crick" in the neck or back
5. Useful for rheumatoid arthritis
6. Prepares the patient for a cold treatment

12. HOT SITZ BATH

General Considerations

1. A full length bathtub may be used. The water should cover the hips and come up onto the abdomen. The feet and hands may be placed in the water, or may be kept out by propping them on the side of the tub.
2. If a tub just large enough for the patient to sit in can be secured, a foot tub with water two to three degrees hotter than the sitz bath may be used in conjunction with the sitz.
3. Use a cold compress to the forehead.
4. A dry sheet may be used to cover the patient and tub if necessary for comfort and protection.
5. The duration of the bath is three to eight minutes for a tonic treatment, or 20-45 minutes for a regular or sedative treatment.
6. A thirty second cold shower, bath, or cold water pour may be used at the end of the bath.

7. The hot sitz bath should be used as a unit with the cold compress to the forehead and the hot foot bath, everything being well prepared ahead of time.
8. As described above, this treatment is remedial, but may be used also as a hygienic measure for the daily program.

Contraindications

1. Extreme obesity with clumsiness
2. Circulatory problems (see contraindications in Hot Foot Bath).

Indications

1. Dysmenorrhea
2. Hemorrhoids and fissures
3. Bladder and prostate inflammation
4. Folliculitis or other skin problems in the perineal region or on the buttocks
5. Salpingitis, oophoritis, pelvic inflammatory disease, cellulitis
6. Atonic constipation
7. Postpartum perineal care

13. SHORT COLD BATH

Indication

1. Most metabolic and degenerative conditions for which fever treatments are used (This treatment is usually as effective as fever, but is not as pleasant for the patient).
2. Multiple sclerosis
3. Colds and influenza
4. Typhoid and other fevers
5. Scarlet fever
6. Rheumatic fever
7. Malaria
8. Lupus erythematosus

Contraindications

1. Chilled patient (very important)
2. Extreme fear of chilling
3. Temperature rising and patient feels chilly (precede with a fever treatment for a few minutes, or a hot foot bath).

Procedure

1. Fill the tub with water from 55° to 90°, or adjust the shower similarly if it is to be substituted.
2. Friction or percussion is always given with the bath. If the shower is used, a forceful, heavy, large drop shower into which one quickly plunges is more easily tolerated than a delicate, fine spray that gradually covers the body. Give the patient a coarse washcloth or mitts for each hand, or a luffa sponge. The therapist may use a moderately coarse brush.
3. Briefly bathe the face in cold water and dry briskly before the bath begins. A brush massage of the entire body may precede the cold plunge.
4. Assist the patient to enter the bath and begin rubbing immediately.
5. The time varies from a brief plunge to 20 or more minutes. Typhoid is treated at 75° to 90° for 15 minutes. It is well to give the first bath in a series at 90° and reduce it 5° each day. At colder temperatures (55° to 75°) the entire treatment lasts for 30 to 180 seconds.
6. Keep the blood flowing briskly to the skin by constant rubbing. Have a second attendant take pulse and temperature readings frequently if a bath longer than 3 minutes is used.
7. Finish the bath with a brisk rubdown using a dry coarse towel. Reaction time in bed is 30 to 60 minutes.

14. SALT GLOW

The salt glow is a stimulant type of special massage which can be used for a number of conditions. It is a very pleasant treatment if given properly.

Indications

1. Epilepsy
2. General tonic
3. Chronic illness of any kind
4. Stimulant for muscles, nerves, or skin
5. Cancer and other debilitating diseases

Contraindications

1. Patient who cannot stand or sit
2. Skin rashes, or open, weeping lesions
3. The same as for a hot foot bath

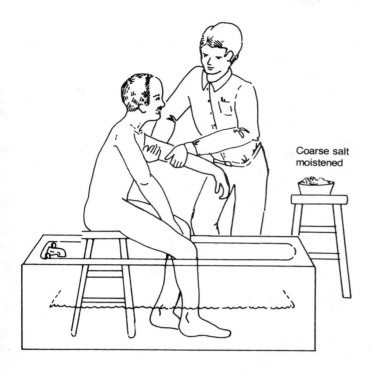

Coarse salt
moistened

Procedure

1. Stand the patient (or seat a weak patient on a stool) in an ordinary bath tub.
2. Put about one-half cup of salt in a quart size dish, plastic or steel. Ordinary table salt may be used, but a coarser grade is much preferred.
3. Moisten the salt thoroughly, just enough to make the grains stick together, but not enough to dissolve the salt.
4. Use enough hot water in the tub to cover the ankles of the person.
5. Take approximately 1 tablespoon of the moistened salt in the hands and distribute between the two palms. Take an extremity and use a brisk upward movement with one hand while making a downward movement with the other hand; quickly alternate and give a friction massage to the entire extremity, the patient holding the extremity stiff. Move to the next extremity, and friction all four extremities. Then friction the back, using an up-and-down rubbing motion, alternating with the two hands until the entire back has been thoroughly covered. Proceed with a similar motion over the chest and abdomen, if desired. Have the patient sit on a stool to elevate one foot if that helps facilitate the application to the thighs, legs and ankles.
6. Use a cool shower or a pail pour to cleanse the skin at the end. The water should be at a pleasant tem-

perature. Rub the skin vigorously during rinsing, the patient assisting.

7. Use a vigorous friction motion with the towel to dry the patient.

15. HOT WATER BOTTLE

Hot water bottles can be purchased from a drug store, or a plastic detergent bottle or any empty plastic bottle may be used as a hot water bottle. Several sizes may be kept on hand to fit in several angles of the body, such as under the chin, by the waist, or behind the knee.

These simple devices have many uses, and when properly used can bring great relief. They should be standard equipment in every well-run home. Yet often a drug will be taken which risks injury of the health for all future time, when a hot water bottle would have been even more effective, more economical, and entirely safe.

Fill the hot water bottle about half to two-thirds full with water at about 135° to 150°. Test the stopper for leakage. Be certain to expel the air when the bottle is being filled. Wrap it well in a cloth or put it in a pillowcase; place it on the area to be treated. Great care must be used to protect paralyzed patients or those whose skin is not sensitive to heat.

Use a hot water bottle for any pain, including that in teeth or in the abdomen. All skeletal aches and pains, including fresh sprains, may be properly treated with a hot water bottle, contrary to the former belief that only ice packs should be used. Hot water bottles may be used to augment a heating compress or fomentation.

When storing the hot water bottle hang it upside down on a hook with the stopper out. The stopper can be attached to the bottom of the bag with a twist tie. Do not leave it doubled or folded for storage.

16. HEATING PAD

The same remarks can be made for the benefits of electric heating pads as for hot water bottles. They are useful in peptic ulcers, bursitis, backache, arthritis, any skeletal pain, chest congestion, asthma, and many other conditions. For coughs, lay the heating pad in the bed at the level of the shoulder blades. Often the derivative effect of the heat on the skin will abolish the cough. For afflictions of the perineum or seat area, a heating pad can be placed in a chair and the patient seated on it. For skeletal or back problems, a heating pad can be placed in the bed and the patient laid upon it. It may be wrapped around an extremity, folded and wrapped about the neck, or draped over a shoulder. For many types of pain or discomfort, no other measure need be used.

To use an electric device such as a heating pad with

wet packs, simply cover the heating pad with a large garbage bag for protection. If a radio is plugged into the same outlet with the heating pad, and turned on low to a silent area on the dial, static will notify one of a short in the electric circuit before a serious problem such as a fire would arise.

When used over a wet compress the same effect is obtained as with fomentations, the main difference being inability to control the applications as well.

17. HEAT LAMP

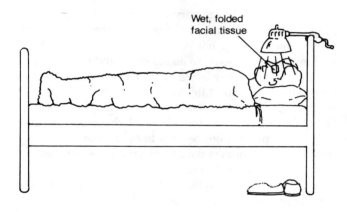

Wet, folded facial tissue

An ordinary shop lamp obtained at a hardware store can serve nicely as a heat lamp. The lamp can be clamped to the head of the bed or to a makeshift arm from the bedboard so that it may be suspended over various parts of the body. Many conditions are best treated by a heat lamp: (1) When the nasal passages are swollen with a cold and sleep is impossible, simply fix a heat lamp with a 100 watt bulb in a position about two inches from the nose. Two bottle caps or squares of tissue moistened for weight and molding, can be laid over the eyes to protect them from the brightness of the lamp. The nasal passages open up as by magic. (2) An earache is best treated by a heat lamp with a 100 watt bulb. Even small babies will usually lie perfectly still when the idea is communicated and the pain relief from the heat is experienced. (3) Perineal care in the postpartum period can be augmented by the use of a heat lamp. When there is burning and discomfort in the perineal area, the heat lamp is without peer in giving relief simply and without an assistant. Especially when used after a hot tub sitz it is very soothing and healing.

The average treatment with a heat lamp is 20 to 30 minutes, but a person with an earache may get several hours' relief and sleep with its use, where rest without it may be impossible.

Infrared bulb—The heat from the infrared bulb is much more intense than the electric light bulb and can be used for special situations. In post partum cases with stinging or discomfort of the perineal structures, the infrared bulb may be used, although generally the common incandescent electric light bulb is quite sufficient, and delivers all the heat the patient can tolerate. Use the infrared bulb according to the instructions on the package.

A shop lamp with a screen wire shield over a globe is ideal for this kind of treatment. A shop lamp which will satisfy all needs can be purchased for a few dollars.

Ultraviolet light—The ultraviolet light can be used for patients who need daily sun bathing, but because of weather or patient conditions cannot get out-of-doors. Use the ultraviolet lamp according to the package instructions.

18. CASTOR OIL PACKS

Equipment

1. Flannel cloth
2. Plastic sheet
3. Electric heating pad
4. Bath towel
5. Two safety pins
6. Six ounces of castor oil

Procedure

First, prepare a folded soft flannel cloth (preferably wool flannel, but cotton flannel is satisfactory), two to four thicknesses about ten inches in width and twelve to fourteen inches in length. This is the size needed after folding for abdominal applications. Pour some castor oil onto the cloth. This is done without soiling if the plastic sheet is under the cloth. Make sure the cloth is wet but not dripping with castor oil. Apply the cloth to the skin.

Next, lay the plastic sheet over the soaked flannel cloth. Then place a heating pad, turned up first to "medium," then to "high" if tolerated. The heating process may be assisted by wrapping a towel, folded lengthwise, around the entire area, and fastening it with safety pins. The pack should remain in place for one to eight hours.

The skin should be cleansed afterward by using soda water prepared by adding one teaspoon of baking soda to one pint of cool water. Dip a cloth into the soda water and rub the skin briskly until it is thoroughly cleansed. Keep the flannel pack in a plastic container for future use. It need not be discarded after one application.

Frequency of use: Seven consecutive days for the

first week, every other day the second week, and three times a week the third week.

Indications

1. Peptic ulcer (Apply over the lower chest and upper abdomen.)
2. Colitis
3. Cancer
4. Prostate or female pelvic problems (Apply to low abdomen, groins, medial thighs and seat area.)
5. Arthritis
6. Appendicitis, as a poultice over the right flank, groin, and lower abdomen

19. DOUCHES (VAGINAL IRRIGATIONS)

Douching is probably never necessary for women with normal vaginal secretions. Pregnant women should not douche. In vaginitis or cervicitis, however, it may be desirable to wash out the vagina with a cleansing stream of water or douche solution. Do not rush the procedure; allow 5-10 minutes.

From a pharmacy obtain a douche kit, including a 2 quart bag, plastic tubing with a clasp for starting and stopping flow, and a hard plastic douche nozzle with holes around all sides. The bag usually has a hole near the top which can be threaded onto a clothes hanger so the bag can be suspended from a position not more than about 2 feet above the hips. It may be hung on a chairback, towel rack, shower or soapcup rod, or it may be laid on the edge of the bathtub.

Assume a convenient position for the douche, lying or sitting in the tub at about a 45° angle. Sitting upright prevents a proper flow of the douche solution into all the crevices and folds of the vagina. Bend the knees, spread apart, and insert the nozzle. Alternate positions are sitting in a shower stall or on the commode leaning back as far as possible. A low stool may be used to raise the feet off the floor a few inches.

Release the clasp and allow the solution to flow into the vagina. To cleanse the many folds and creases, fill the vagina with fluid by folding the lips of the vulva around the nozzle with the thumb and forefinger until sufficient solution has distended the vagina and a sense of fullness or pressure is experienced over the bladder. Shut off the clasp and hold the solution for as long as required to count slowly to 15. Let the fluid gush out. Repeat this procedure until all of the solution is used.

Clean the equipment by washing with soap and water. Rinse well and hang it up with the clasp open to encourage drainage and drying of the interior of the tube.

The equipment may be sterilized by a solution of lysol water. Use 1 tablespoon of lysol to a quart of water. Fill the bag and tubing and allow to set for 15 minutes. Rinse well and dry as described.

Select an appropriate solution from the list at the end of this description. Start a treatment series using three hot douches daily for three days for most ordinary infections, then dropping to two douches daily for three days, then once daily for thirty days.

Generally the douche is not used during pregnancy. Cervicitis and vaginitis occurring in the pregnant woman are treated with hot foot baths, perineal hygiene, all-cotton panties, and showers rather than tub baths which might allow the contaminated bath water to enter the vagina. Hot foot baths increase the circulation of blood to the vagina, cervix, and entire pelvic area. This simple treatment may be done safely. Absorption occurs more readily from the vagina than from the gastrointestinal tract making any cream or suppository used during pregnancy a hazard to the developing infant.

Douche Solutions

1. Hot water. The commonest and most useful solution for vaginal irrigation is merely hot water, 2-4 quarts at 105° to 110°.
2. Vinegar. For a vinegar douche, use one to four tablespoons of any kind of vinegar to each quart of hot water. For one treatment use two quarts of solution. This is the standard douche solution and should be selected for all ordinary infections and cleansing. It should be used for trichomonas, but not for monilia or thrush. The vagina is normally quite acid, and the use of an acid douche solution helps to restore the normal pH of the vagina, which may be altered by an infection.
3. Baking soda. For the baking soda douche use one teaspoon of baking soda to each quart of water. For one treatment use two quarts of solution. This solution is most applicable for monilia or yeast infections, and should always be tried when vinegar is not successful within a reasonable treatment period.
4. Garlic. One clove of garlic may be blended in one quart of boiling water, cooled, and strained if desired, for a garlic douche solution. Use one quart of solution for a treatment. Use the garlic solution raw, or cooked for 1-5 minutes if the tissues are very tender and sensitive. Use it for infections that are resistant to the usual treatments. It often brings remarkable results in vaginitis.
5. Styptic. For a styptic douche use comfrey or golden seal, two heaping tablespoons of tea leaves to one quart of water. Steep for 15 minutes and strain. Use

this douche for bleeding surfaces such as cervicitis or vaginitis.

6. Charcoal. One tablespoon of charcoal may be added to a quart of water to make a charcoal douche solution for infections, ulcers, and viral diseases.

7. Lysol. Lysol, a 2.7% product of phenol, water and soap, with other phenols and alcohols and inert material, is a good antiseptic. Use one-half to one teaspoon of lysol to one quart of water at 100° to 105°. Mix the solution well. Lysol tends to cause a sensitivity reaction in some individuals. Should sensitivity, rash, or burning begin, immediately stop the use of lysol and it should clear up promptly. This douche may be used to combat heavy bacterial infections of the cervix and vagina, and in postpartum care. The same solution may be used for ordinary antiseptic perineal care, and for deodorizing the perineum, underarms, feet, or skin lesions that develop odor. Simply pour a small paper cupful of the solution over the perineum or skin lesions, or sponge the underarms with a tissue saturated with the solution. It is a good deodorant, but watch for sensitivities.

20. ENEMAS

Enemas are useful for cleansing the bowel and preparing the bowel to take an active role in ridding the body of toxic substances or infection. Enemas given hot or cold can help control the flow of blood to the abdomen and to the structures of the bowel. Cold water enemas retard the flow of blood to the abdomen and produce retrostasis of blood in the legs, chest and head. Hot water enemas encourage blood flow to the abdomen. Diarrhea, intestinal parasites, ulcerative colitis and other bowel problems can be treated with a hot enema. The cold enema can be used to treat pelvic congestion in acute pelvic inflammatory disease, and other congestive disorders inside the abdomen. When fighting pain anywhere in the body remember that the enema can be used to relieve pain, even in a distant part such as the head or a broken bone. Both hot and cold enemas stimulate the reflexive action of the body; therefore to promote cleansing of the bowel use hot or cold water; for a retention enema, use a lukewarm solution.

The injudicious use of enemas in children can result in bowel perforation and rupture. The rupture is secondary to elevated hydrostatic pressure from the enema. Patients with chronic constipation or congenital diseases are especially likely to absorb large amounts of water from enemas. Occasionally a direct injury results in perforation. One fourteen month old girl was given four tap water and two soapsuds enemas by her parents following a fall from a bicycle. The child died from low salt level in the blood because of absorption of water into the blood from the colon and rupture of the transverse colon.[95]

Procedure

Select the proper solution for the enema from the list at the end of this description. Put the water or solution in a two-quart enema bag and expel air from the tubing. Adjust the height of the bag for the desired rapidity of delivery from hip high to shower curtain rod height, hanging the bag on a shower curtain hook. The rapid injection of enema water can set off a reflex to defecate that the patient finds hard to control. For the enema, sit on the commode (debilitated persons or a child may be placed in a bathtub, stopper removed). The enema water should be held a few minutes before releasing it, if possible. The enema may be repeated in an adult for additional cleansing if the first enema is not clear at the end.

Retention Enema

For the person who cannot take fluids by mouth, the retention enema will in most instances be able to supply the entire water needs of the person. Simply place 8 to 16 ounces (1 to 2 cups) of lukewarm water or saline (1 teaspoon of salt to 2 cups water) in an enema bag and allow it to run slowly into the rectum. A specially prepared mineral replacement solution may be used (see fluid administration section). Lubricate the nozzle well, as repeated insertions, if not done gently, can be quite irritating to the anus and produce painful fissures. The patient can direct you in a gentle insertion if inquiry is made. Repeat the fluid injection every two to four hours for a person not taking fluids in any other way, until two quarts per day have been absorbed. More can be used in a sweating or dehydrated person.

Enema Solutions

1. Water. Use plain hot water at 104 to 110°.
2. Charcoal. Dissolve one to five tablespoons of charcoal in two quarts of water. For a retention enema, use one tablespoon of charcoal powder to 8 ounces of lukewarm water, pushed in gently. If a reflex elimination urge develops, the buttocks can be pinched together until the urge to eliminate passes. Use the charcoal retention enema for any toxic state such as snakebite, kidney failure, or drug ingestion; or for inflammations and infections as ulcerative colitis, inflamed fissures or hemorrhoids.
3. Golden seal. Prepare golden seal solution as directed

above under douche solutions. Most herb teas can be used double strength as a cleansing enema, or regular strength as a retention enema.

4. Oil. Use one to four tablespoons of olive oil in four to six ounces of warm water as a retention enema, or to soften and lubricate impacted feces.

5. Starch enema. First give a cleansing enema of 2 quarts of plain hot water. Then prepare a thin paste of starch (use kitchen cornstarch) in one to two ounces of cool water. Pour the paste into 1 pint of hot water. Allow to cool and inject into the rectum with a bag or bulb syringe. The starch enema is used to stop diarrhea or to relieve irritation.

21. HEATING COMPRESS, MOIST ABDOMINAL BANDAGE, WET GIRDLE

The heating compress is an application of a cold compress so applied and covered that there occurs an initial cooling with retrostasis which lasts about five minutes, followed by warming up and an increase in circulation. The compress is applied cold, but heats up through the reaction of the body against the cold. Then the heat produced is carefully captured and used to increase the temperature of the tissues.

Indications

The heating compress may be applied to the neck for a sore throat, to the chest for coughs, to the abdomen for constipation or abdominal pain, and to any body part for pain or infection, even to the sinuses by using a knit cap to hold the compress in place on the upper face. Use at night around the abdomen and back for sedation, chronic active hepatitis, backache, ulcerative colitis, chronic indigestion, and chronic stomach problems. Use on the feet for a cold.

Equipment (See table on page 57)

1. One to two thicknesses of cotton or linen, or two to four thicknesses of cotton gauze cut to fit the area to be covered, about 2 x 14 x 20″ for throat.

2. A plastic covering about 3″ x 14″ for throat, or large enough to cover the wet cotton piece by at least one-half inch on all sides.

3. Wool flannel or synthetic material cut to fit the area and large enough to cover all of the cotton and plastic. A piece 3″ x 4″ x 34″ will wrap around the neck twice. A wool or synthetic scarf or sports sock will suffice.

4. Moist abdominal binder. Use a strip of woolen or

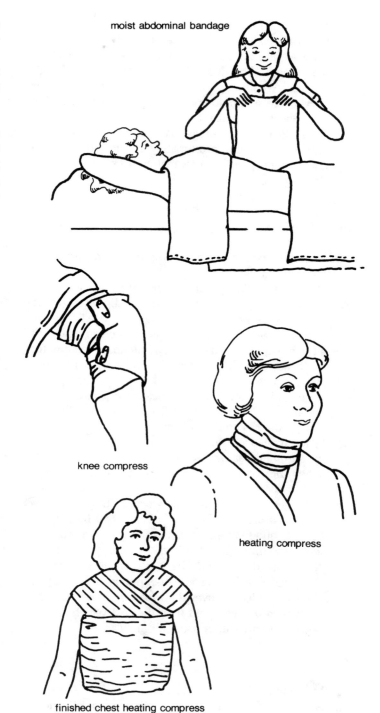

moist abdominal bandage

knee compress

heating compress

finished chest heating compress

Four types of heating compresses:
1. *Chest heating compress*
2. *Moist abdominal bandage*
3. *Throat heating compress*
4. *Heating compress for knee*

The heating compress has many uses: pain, infection, inflammation, swelling, cough, and many others. It should be used more frequently than is customary as a home remedy.

acrylic material such as wool flannel or men's suiting material made from a grade of wool not as stiff or thick as felt, but relatively thin and easily workable. The length should be 55 inches and the width 12 inches. A cotton piece used under the woolen or acrylic piece should measure approximately 50" x 10". Short strips may be sewed together.

5. Chest heating compress. Woolen or acrylic piece should measure approximately 10" x 100" and the cotton underpiece approximately 9" x 100".
6. Safety pins.
7. Cold or ice water.

Procedure

1. Wring the cotton or linen compress from cold water and mold it over the part.
2. Cover it completely with plastic, fitting it snugly, but not tight enough to cause discomfort. Be certain there are no portions of the wet cotton exposed. For the chest a large plastic bag such as a dry cleaning bag or a trash bag may be used. Cut a hole in the bottom for the head, and in the sides for the head and arms. Wear it as a pullover sweater.
3. Wrap and pin the wool flannel securely over the first two layers. Pin any loose fabric into darts so that the end product is smooth fitting.
4. Leave it on from half an hour to overnight, or between other treatments.
5. When the compress is removed, rub the skin which was under the compress with cold water or alcohol.
6. Heating compresses may be worn in the daytime by wearing a nice scarf instead of the wool flannel.
7. For a heating compress to the feet use two pairs of socks, the inner pair wet in cold water. Next, put ordinary bread bags over the wet socks to hold in the moisture of each wet sock; then put on a second pair of socks, rolled on over the bread bags. Be sure the feet warm up well, and then the feet will be a few degrees warmer than usual all night.

Effects

1. Mild tonic (if short application).
2. Sedative (if long duration), secondary to mild heating.
3. Increases deep local blood flow by reflexive action. This treatment to the feet acts to reflexively increase the circulation in the upper respiratory passages and the pelvic area, similar to a hot foot bath.
4. Mild local sweating (especially if covered and augmented by a hot water bottle, heat lamp or heating pad).

5. Relaxation of muscles and blood vessels locally.
6. Pain relief.
7. Infections: sore throat, cough, boils, cellulitis, abdominal distress, whooping cough, croup, pneumonia, constipation.

Precautions

1. Wring dry enough not to drip.
2. When the patient does not soon warm up the wet compress, use a heat lamp, fomentation, heating pad or hot water bottle. Elderly, thin, or debilitated patients may have difficulty warming up the compress, especially if it is large.
3. Avoid chilling.
4. Be sure the wet compress is completely covered by plastic.
5. Apply snugly, but not so tight as to cut off the circulation or limit joint motion.
6. If worn continuously day and night, the wet compress should be changed every 8 hours, and one hour allowed for the skin to dry, to avoid a dermatitis from continuous moisture on the skin.

22. WET DRESSINGS (MOIST SOAKS) See also the Cold Compress

Water is the active ingredient in many expensive commercial lotions, rubs and soaps. The evaporation of water from the skin surface results in vasoconstriction, relief of itching, and congestion and the removal of crusts. An infected dermatitis is effectively treated with wet dressings. Another purpose of a wet dressing is to keep moist an area of skin that would otherwise crack or dry and prevent healing. Squeeze a small linen towel from the proper solution, leaving it very moist but not actually dripping. Cotton pajamas, leotards, long-sleeved shirts or cotton gauze can serve on large areas as wet dressings. After the pajamas are wrung out until damp and placed on the skin, cover them with dry pajamas. Never place plastic over a wet dressing as it prevents the necessary evaporation. Allow the moisture to evaporate slowly over a 4-6 hour period. The dressings are then completely removed and fresh dressings replaced. Boil all cloths used and sun dry if possible before reusing. Maximum benefit occurs at 48 to 72 hours, after which continued application of wet dressings is of little benefit.

The commonest wetting agent for wet dressings is plain water. Saline may be used over the eyes or elsewhere. Boric acid solution, 1 teaspoon to a pint of water, is good for the perineum and most other areas. Golden seal tea may be used for its astringent action.

23. STEAM INHALATION, MEDICATED OR PLAIN

Equipment

1. Vaporizor or kettle with hot water.
2. Newspaper cone or umbrella and sheet
3. Hot plate if needed
4. Bedside stand or chair
5. Medication: a few drops of eucalyptus oil or wintergreen oil, one to two tablespoons of dried or fresh mint leaves per pint of water

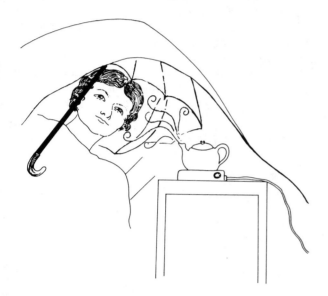

Procedure

1. Fill the vaporizor or kettle with hot water, add medication if desired, and set on a bedside stand or chair.
2. Set an umbrella on the chair or bedside stand, and drape a sheet over it to form a tent. By lying on one side of the bed, the patient can arrange to put his head under the side of the tent and breathe the steam.
3. If desirable, cover the kettle outlet with a cone and direct the steam toward the patient.
4. Continue for one-half to one hour, two to three times a day or more.
5. The cone is not essential in a small closed room.

Effects

1. Warming and soothing for the respiratory tract
2. Relief of nasal and lung congestion, laryngitis or coughs
3. Increased blood flow to the respiratory tree

4. Secretions made more loose and alkaline, and easier to expectorate

Precautions

1. Check water level often in the kettle.
2. Avoid burning patients or setting bedding on fire.
3. Persons with severely compromised cardiovascular systems or congestive heart failure may find air laden with heavy fog hard to breathe.

24. COLD MITTEN FRICTION

Equipment

1. Two or more towels
2. Friction mitts; may use a washcloth wrapped around the hand if mitts are unavailable. However, mitts are easy to make by simply sewing along the sides and one end of a folded washcloth.
3. Pail of cold water 50° to 60° or less

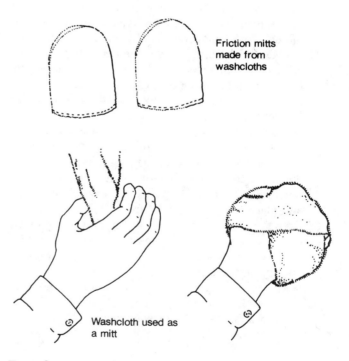

Friction mitts made from washcloths

Washcloth used as a mitt

Procedure

1. Expose right arm. Place one towel folded in half under the right shoulder, and a second one under the arm. Dip the mitts or washcloth into the cold water and squeeze out the excess. Arrange the mitts on your hands. Use only one hand if washcloth is used.

Catch one corner of the washcloth in the palm, wrap the hand with the washcloth, and catch the other corner in the palm, making a fist covered with the washcloth.

2. Begin at the fingers and work up the arm with a vigorous to-and-fro friction. You may dip the mitts again and repeat the process. If the skin is not pink, give a third frictioning.

3. Quickly remove mitts. Cover the arm with a towel, having the patient grasp the end of the towel in the hand. Rub vigorously over the towel, then wrap the towel around your hand and give a few long quick friction strokes to the whole arm. Rub the part with your bare hand to be sure it is thoroughly dry.

4. Replace the right arm under the sheet, and treat the left arm in the same manner.

5. Expose the chest and abdomen, placing a towel over each arm, tucking it well under the shoulders and sides to prevent chilling the arms.

6. While standing at the bedside facing the patient, with the mitts on your hands, ask the patient to take a deep breath. Give a short to-and-fro friction, first to the chest up the midline, out over the shoulders, down the sides to the bedline, then back to the midline. Go over the surface twice, then quickly dip the mitts in the cold water and repeat. Dry briskly in the same way as for the arms. Cover the chest and abdomen with a towel or sheet and blanket. Avoid injuring the breasts or nipples, or getting the bedclothing wet.

7. Expose the right leg and foot. Bend the knee, place one towel under the thigh and heel lengthwise, another across the upper thigh. Proceed as with the arm. Dry and friction the left lower extremity. Cover.

8. Turn the patient to the prone position, pillow under the lower chest if needed for comfort, arms raised to the level of the head. Expose the back including hips, and place towels as for the front of the body.

9. Give a to-and-fro friction with up and down movements; crosswise movements may also be used over the lower back and hips. Dip the mitts and repeat.

10. To vary the tonic effect, change the intensity and temperature of the water. More water left in the mitts and more friction will give a more vigorous reaction. Coarser mitts or a luffa sponge may be used for greater friction.

Effects

1. Restores tone to blood vessels and muscles: called a "vascular gymnastic"
2. Increases heat production
3. Increases muscular, glandular, and metabolic activities of internal organs

4. Increases phagocytosis and anti-bacterial activities
5. Increases oxidation and elimination of bacterial toxins
6. Produces a general tonic for prevention or treatment of colds, low energy and endurance, poor resistance to infections, tobacco and drug withdrawal, alcoholism, poor circulation, anemia and low thyroid activity

Precautions

1. The room should be at the proper temperature (75° to 80°) and the patient must be warm.
2. Give the friction vigorously with rapid movements.
3. Dry each part thoroughly with or without rubbing, leaving no dampness.
4. Be sure that the bed is not damp after a treatment.
5. If the patient does not have a good reaction, or dislikes the procedure, discontinue it promptly.
6. Avoid frictioning skin lesions or painful areas.

25.   COLD TOWEL RUB

Indications

Same as for cold mitten friction.

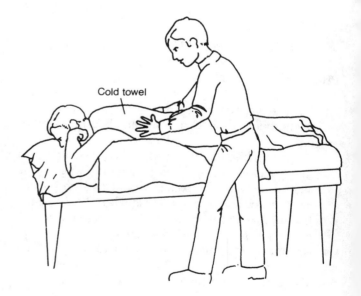

Cold towel

Procedure

1. Dip a towel in cold water and wring lightly. Wrap the towel loosely around the arm lengthwise, the towel end being held firmly in the hand of the patient.
2. Rub the arm briskly on the outside of the cold towel

to achieve a reddening, as in the cold mitten friction. Percussion may be used to promote a more brisk reaction.

3. Dry the arm with a coarse towel using a friction motion. Cover the arm with a sheet and proceed to the next extremity.
4. Treat the back by spreading the cold towel over the back from the shoulders to below the buttocks. Rub as before; dry and cover.
5. The chest and abdomen are treated last. Spread the cold towel from shoulders to groin, having the patient hold the upper corners during the rubbing strokes, which are made from above downward.

Precaution

The patient will lose more heat from the cold towel rub than from the cold mitten friction. This effect should be taken into account in the decision to use this treatment rather than the cold mitten friction.

26. WET SHEET PACK WITH FRICTION RUB, AND HOT EVAPORATING SHEET PACK

The wet sheet to be used in this treatment should not be left too wet, as it tends to change its temperature too rapidly when a lot of water is left in it.

Indications

Use for infections or fevers, mental illness, as a general tonic in chronic illness, chronic eczematoid dermatitis, or other generalized dermatitis.

Contraindications

1. Faintness
2. Phlebitis
3. Boils or open lesions on the skin

Equipment

1. Long cotton bandage to bind a washcloth dipped in cold water to the forehead
2. Tub of hot water
3. Cold water at 60° to 70°, or for the hot sheet pack at 104°
4. Sheet
5. Three pails of water, one at 70°, one at 65°, and one at 60°
6. Coarse towel
7. Four to six clothespins or large safety pins

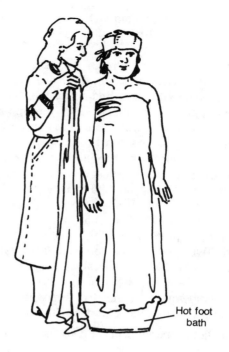

Hot foot bath

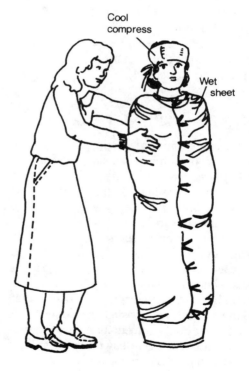

Cool compress

Wet sheet

Procedure

1. Tie a cold compress around the forehead at the beginning of the treatment.
2. Have the patient stand in a hot foot bath if the wet sheet rub is planned.

3. Wring a sheet from cold water at 60 to 70° for a wet sheet rub, or at 104° for the hot evaporating sheet pack.
4. Wind the wet sheet around the patient, beginning under one arm, carry the sheet around the back, under the opposite arm, and across the abdomen. As the wrapping is continued, cover the first shoulder and arm, and tuck it in at the legs and neck. Fasten with clothespins or safety pins.
5. For the wet sheet rub, percuss and friction over the sheet quickly until the sheet becomes warm from the action of the friction and the body heat. At the end of the treatment, which should cover the entire skin surface, pour a pail of water at 70° over the patient. A second pail at 65° and a third pail at 60° should be used. Two operators are best for this treatment. A cool, forceful shower gradually getting cooler can be substituted for the pail pouring if more convenient. The temperature cannot be as easily controlled however. Friction the skin dry with a coarse towel.

In the hot evaporating sheet pack for treating fevers, follow the same basic procedure as for the wet sheet rub except that the hot foot bath is omitted. At the end of the pail pour have the patient sit or lie for a few minutes to reduce the fever, or remove the sheet after one or two minutes and friction dry with a coarse towel, as the condition of the patient permits.

27. HEATING TRUNK PACK

The trunk and hips are wrapped, the extremities excluded. A hot foot bath is given simultaneously. A single blanket is placed crosswise the bed so that the upper edge will reach the armpits and the lower edge will come just below the buttocks when the patient lies on it. A single or double thickness sheeting is next wrung from cold water and laid on the crosswise blanket. It should not extend beyond the edges of the blanket. The patient lies on the wet sheet, arms raised, and the pack begun as for a moist abdominal bandage, by pulling the right side of the wet sheet under the right arm, over the abdomen and tucking it in at the opposite side under the left arm. Place a hot water bottle, fomentation pack, or heating pad covered with a large plastic bag on the first layer of the wet sheet which now covers the abdomen. Subsequently the left side of the wet sheet is wrapped over the patient and tucked in on the other side. Then the blanket is wrapped snugly around the patient and fastened with large pins or clothes pins or simply tucked in. The patient's arms are now brought down and a shirt is put on backward or a sheet and blanket used to cover the patient. General sweating should be produced.

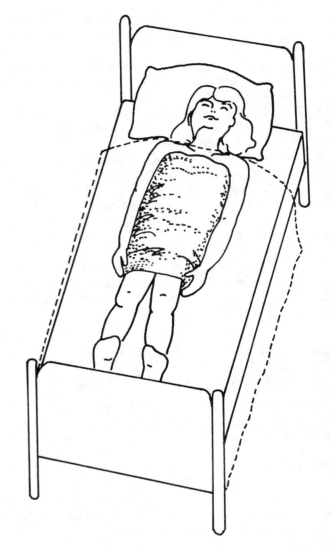

If this treatment is used for persistent nausea and vomiting (as in pregnancy or some peptic ulcers) begin one-half hour before the meal and continue if needed for two to three hours following the meal. This is one of the most effective treatments for digestive disturbances. It promotes gastric secretions, liver activity, and normalizes the motility of the gastrointestinal tract. Gas production is checked. It may also be used for dyspepsia, indigestion, flatulence, chronic congestion of the liver, and reduced gastric motility. For these conditions 20-25 minutes is the usual treatment time.

28. THE HOT HALF BATH: ARTIFICIAL FEVER TREATMENT FOR HOME USE

Fever and hyperthermia are not actually equivalents, but in general use in hydrotherapy one hears the terms "fever treatment," "artificial fever," and "hyperthermia" used interchangeably. Fever is actually an elevated thermoregulatory "set-point" in the hypothalamus. Hyperthermia occurs when the core temperature rises above the "set point." Any degree of artificial elevation of the body temperature with a bath or blanket pack is generally called a "fever treatment," even if the oral temperature goes no higher than 100°.

Procedure (See also Item 2. of this section for institutional use of fever treatments.)

Fill the bathtub with water quite a bit under the hottest that can be tolerated and have the patient lie in the tub, a cushion or folded towel for the head. Record the initial oral temperature. As soon as the patient is settled and adjusted to the hot water, raise the water temperature to the hottest that can be tolerated, 105° to 115°. It is not good to start out at the hottest temperature, as some patients will react to very hot water in the same way as to very cold water, by goose flesh and constriction of blood vessels, not only locally, but at a distance, as in the head.

To convert a half bath to a full bath, and produce a quicker elevation of the temperature, cover the knees and shoulders of the patient with a towel dipped in the hot bath water. By using a dipper or cup, dip water from the bathtub onto the towels to keep all portions of the patient in contact with the hot water.

Put a thermometer in the mouth and check it every five minutes. After about five to six minutes for an adult the temperature should be approximately 100°. At that time, or before if sweating has begun, apply a cold wash cloth wrung from ice water to the forehead. Sponge the face and neck frequently with a cold cloth. Keep the head cool at all times, being especially careful to sponge the face and change the head cloth often when the temperature is over 102°. Remember that cold compresses to the throat make the oral temperature go down, and the body may be hotter than the thermometer indicates. For this reason, a check of the pulse rate should be made periodically. If the pulse goes over 140 or the patient complains of extreme discomfort, you may promptly restore the pulse and body temperature by adding cold water to the bath.

The duration of the treatment may be determined either by time or by temperature. When treating ordinary acute problems such as simple colds, flu, or cricks in the neck or back, it may be well to terminate the bath when the temperature has reached 102° to 103°. For ordinary chronic problems such as persistent cough, eczema, or psoriasis, maintain the mouth temperature at 101° to 103° for 5 to 45 minutes (the serious illnesses require higher temperatures and longer treatment times.), by reducing the water temperature to about 106°. Stabilize the mouth temperature by carefully regulating the water temperature. A small electric fan may be directed toward the face for patient comfort if it does not reduce body temperature. The temperature may be kept up for one to four hours. During the first hour, give only water to drink; after one hour use saline solution made by putting 1 teaspoon of salt in two to four cups of water. Encourage two to four glasses of water or saline per hour.

Finishing the Bath

The treatment should be ended properly for the greatest effectiveness and comfort for the patient. A shower, a cold mitten friction, or an alcohol rub may be used to properly finish the bath. Since much blood will be out at the skin surface, and the fluid lost in sweating may not be entirely replaced by drinking, the internal blood volume may be less than when the person was put in the tub. Therefore a period of faintness may be experienced after a few seconds of standing up. This reaction is one sign of a successful treatment, but may be unpleasant. To avoid this unpleasantness, work fast to prepare the patient for bed.

The bed should be prepared ahead of time by laying a towel to protect the bed, as sweating will continue about 30 minutes. Have the patient stand up in the tub and turn around briefly (10-30 seconds) in a cool or cold shower while briskly rubbing the skin with the hands.[96] If desired, one can pour the remainder of the ice water used to sponge the face over the patient to intensify and prolong the redness, splashing it front and back from the shoulders down, reserving some for the feet. Have the patient lift one foot, and pour the cold water over it, and step from the tub. Then the other foot is lifted from the bath water, and the remaining cold water poured over it. Dry briskly with coarse towels, the patient assisting. When the patient assists there is less likelihood of fainting. Wrap a sheet around the patient and walk immediately to the bed. If the patient feels faint, while continuing to walk, he may bend over to lower the head. Cover with blankets if it is desirable to continue the fever. Protect the pillow with a towel and wrap a second towel around the neck to catch the sweat. After 30-60 minutes of reaction time, sweating will have ceased, a brief neutral shower should be taken for cleansing and readjustment of the temperature.

Continue to keep the head cool and to administer water after the transfer to bed, until the mouth temperature is below 100°. For the short bath and those at low mouth temperatures, 102° and below, the bath can be easily self-administered by a vigorous and healthy person.

For small children use a rule of thumb for time and temperature. If the bath water is not above 103° no injury can be done to the child even if the time of the bath is prolonged to 10 or 15 minutes. At bath temperatures above 105°, and especially near 110°, use three minutes for babies up to three years of age, and one minute for each year of age after age three. Have a stopwatch or reliable person as a timekeeper for small babies, to avoid overheating. Remember that the temperature rises more rapidly if a fever is already present, and a lower bath temperature should be used. If the oral temperature is already 103° or above, use a 3 minute bath only, for children over age 3; use less time for infants, only sufficient to induce muscle relaxation and deep breathing. Adjust the bath temperature to 106° if the rectal temperature is 103°; have the bath water at 105° if rectal temperature is 104°; adjust the bath at 104° if rectal temperature is 105°. Finish off the bath with a brief cold water pour and a brisk rubbing with a towel to increase the action of the skin. (See chart "Hot Baths for Fevers.")

Effects of the Hot Half Bath

1. Stimulates the immune mechanisms in infections; raises white blood cell count, increases the vigor of phagocytosis
2. Reduces fever by reversing heat conservation and initiating heat dissipation processes
3. Eliminates toxins by sweating
4. Relaxes spastic muscles of cricks in the neck and back
5. Invariably reduces blood pressure
6. Quiets diarrhea
7. Tends to stabilize a disturbed mind
8. Almost invariably produces sleep in small children; if mild and long, is sedative for adults
9. Leaves a sense of well-being after fluid equilibrium is re-established

29. THE NEUTRAL BATH

The neutral bath is given in the same way as the hot half bath, except that the water of the bath is around 94° to 98°. Except in mental or neurological diseases there is no need to sponge the face or forehead with cold water, as sweating is minimal or absent. It may be maintained from ten minutes to several hours, even all day for a disturbed person, or for intractable itching.

The benefits of the neutral bath result from the use of water so employed as to be absolutely non-irritating, without mechanical friction or percussion, and of such a temperature as to shield the body from the continued ex-

citation resulting from contact of the skin with the clothing, constantly changing temperature, force of movement and various other disturbing influences. The nerve centers, as a result of a total lack of excitation, are afforded an opportunity to accumulate a store of energy so that a recuperation, sedation, and energizing may occur.

The type of termination of the bath will depend on the effect desired and on the next activity the person expects to do. If the person is going to work, use a cold mitten friction and brisk rubdown. If one is going to bed to sleep, blot the skin dry, dress in soft clothing, and move slowly so as not to excite or stimulate the nerves.

Indications

1. Insomnia
2. Agitation
3. Itching
4. Depression
5. Any mental illness
6. Lowering of blood pressure in acute hypertension

30. THE CONTINUOUS BATH, HAMMOCK BATH

Definition

The continuous bath consists of a bathtub full of water at neutral temperature, the patient remaining in the bath for hours, days, weeks, or months as the case may require. Hebra is reported to have kept a case of pemphigus in the continuous bath for four years with much benefit. Bernard Fantus reported a very offensive ischio-rectal abscess which had broken into the scrotum and was extending upward on the body in all directions. After becoming adapted to the bath, the patient was so relieved of discomfort and so happy to be rid of the odor that he objected to being removed even once a day for cleansing the tub, and the rubbing of his skin with petrolatum. After 10 days and nights in the bath the condition had cleared sufficiently to permit ordinary dressing. The patient left the hospital in about a month, practically healed!

Indications

1. Constant removal of profuse or offensive exudates from abscesses, sloughing cancers, foul-smelling urinary or fecal fistulae, or extensive gangrene
2. Pemphigus
3. Itching

4. Sedation in agitated mental patients, mania or delirium tremens
5. Extensive burns
6. Pain and paresthesias
7. Spasms

Procedure

1. Everything possible must be done to make the patient comfortable in the tub. With carpenter's clamps or strong hooks suspend a hammock or sheet within the tub in such a way that it will clear the bottom of the tub when the patient is lying on it. A rubber pillow should be provided for the head and one for the heels. If possible, leave the feet out of the water to avoid swelling and wrinkling of the skin.
2. Rub the skin with vaseline or lanolin once daily when the patient is removed for thorough bathing with soap and soft brush. The patient should exercise a bit at this time. The tub is also cleansed with soap and brush, and an antiseptic applied in cases of infection. After thorough rinsing, the water is replaced and the patient again enters the tub.[98]

31. THE SHAMPOO

A shampoo can be given to a patient while lying crosswise in bed. Place a plastic, such as a shower curtain, under the patient's shoulders. Towels and pillows are so arranged on the edge of the bed to form a sort of trough from a pillow under the patient's shoulders to the edge. A tub or large pan is placed on the floor beside the bed. The plastic is allowed to trail off the edge of the bed into the tub. The shampoo should be diluted somewhat with water and used to wet the patient's scalp and hair. A lather should be worked up, using extra water from a bottle that can be easily manipulated. Rinsing should be done from a large pitcher set on a stool or chair beside the bed. Use one or two soapings, rinse well, towel dry, and wrap with a second dry towel.

Clear away the materials, making certain the patient's bed is dry—if not, cover all moist places with a dry towel. With patient in the same position as for the shampoo, blow-dry hair with an electric hair drier.

Golden seal tea, double strength, may be used as a final rinse when treating eczema of the scalp. When treating impetigo, following the final rinsing, work a charcoal paste into the scalp, allow it to remain for 4 hours, and repeat the shampoo.

32. PARAFFIN BATH

This is an effective way to deliver heat to a painful body part. The internal temperature of the part is elevated, relieving pain and inducing healing. It is a pleasant treatment and leaves the skin soft and smooth.

Indications

1. Arthritis
2. Bruises
3. Bursitis
4. Gout
5. Pain
6. Sprains
7. Strains
8. Tennis elbow

Contraindications

1. Skin infections
2. Hardening of arteries (precludes treatment of the lower extremities)
3. Reduced sensation in the part
4. Dermatitis from paraffin

Equipment

1. Double boiler
2. Five pounds of paraffin
3. Mineral oil
4. Bath thermometer

Procedure

1. Use a large double boiler or slow cooker of sufficient size to accommodate the hands and wrists.
2. Fill the inner chamber of the cooker about two-thirds full with commercial paraffin such as Parowax. Add sufficient mineral oil to comprise by measure or weight up to 20% the total mixture (1/2 to 1 pint of mineral oil to five pounds of paraffin).
3. Obtain from a department store a dairy thermometer capable of registering up to 150°.
4. Melt the paraffin in the inner chamber of the double boiler, usually an hour or more. When the paraffin in the inner chamber is at a temperature of 125° to 135°, immerse the hands and immediately withdraw them, repeating several times in order to obtain a thick glove of solidified paraffin. Finally place the hands in

the paraffin and keep them there for 30 minutes. At the end of this time, peel off the gloves and replace them in the cooker. This treatment should be taken once daily.

5. The paraffin bath may be followed by massage and exercise for the hands.

6. The paraffin bath to the hands usually causes the patient to perspire profusely. Therefore, it is desirable to follow it by a thirty minute reaction period in bed and a warm bath or shower for cleansing and readjustment of body temperature.

33. MUD BATHS

Tests have shown that extracts from clay and other earth samples have antibacterial properties and exhibit features of attaching toxins in somewhat the same fashion as charcoal. A test animal, the dog, was put in mud baths and showed great metabolic changes without injuring the dog in any way. The functions of the heart and kidneys, and the heat-regulating centers remained wholly undisturbed. There was a significant decrease in total acidity of the urine, regarded to be favorable. A summary of the results of one experiment follows: (1) the protracted mud baths at 39° C. had a powerful stimulating effect on metabolism, absorption of inflammatory masses, and promotion of regeneration of tissues, without injuring the system; (2) blood formation was stimulated; (3) the urine was alkalinized; (4) the excretion of chlorides by the kidneys was increased.[99]

An experiment done on four healthy men between the ages of 21 and 52 revealed that after mud extract baths, the skin temperatures were higher than after pure water baths. It was interpreted that the mud extract baths

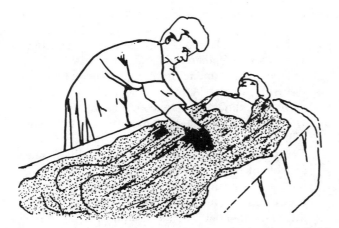

Spread a shower curtain on a cot or in a bathtub, and "ice" the patient with mud, similar to a popular beach activity with sand.

improved blood circulation in the skin and consequently improved heat absorption during the mud extract bath.

Sweat elicited by sweat-producing measures always contains uric acid. Subjects submitted to a daily hot mud pack for a period of two weeks or more eliminated considerable amounts of uric acid through the skin. It was reported that sometimes the percentage of uric acid in the sweat reached a value equal to or exceeding that in the blood. Apparently the skin has the faculty of extracting uric acid from the blood.[93] [94] [95]

Indications

1. Infections, both superficial and deep
2. Pain
3. Swelling
4. Arthritis, gout, sciatica, neuritis
5. Kidney failure with retention of wastes
6. Fluid retention in liver failure, sarcoidosis and other conditions
7. Cancer (for pain, toxin absorption, reduction of swelling)
8. All the indications of charcoal
9. Lupus erythematosus
10. Eczema, skin rashes, poison ivy, other dermatological diseases

Equipment and Materials

1. A tub: an old bathtub set in the sun in a sheltered area is ideal. (If this ideal cannot be achieved, use a large plastic sheet placed in the bed over a trough of folded blankets, laid in the bed in such a fashion as to make a kind of ridge around the outside edges of the trough. See illustration.)
2. Clay obtained after removing the topsoil (Ideally, clay contains no sand or humus, and never pebbles.)

Procedure

1. Put several buckets of clay, about 100 pounds or more, in the bathtub or correspondingly less for the trough in bed.
2. Mix in sufficient hot, warm, or cool water to make a good quality mud about the consistency of soft butter. Use the temperature that best suits the case.
3. The patient sits in the tub and dips the mud to cover all parts of the body, even the face. From time to time the mud is dipped up onto the skin surface to refresh the applications.

If the trough method is used, let the patient lie on the plastic and cover the entire body with several buckets of thick mud, thick enough to make an "icing" about one-half to two-thirds of an inch thick, cover with a plastic sheet and blankets if necessary.

4. The length of the treatment varies with the need—from 20 minutes to 4-6 hours.

5. The mud can be used for several baths, usually about three, before being discarded.

6. When the time is up, the patient shakes off the excess mud, takes a cleansing shower or treatment bath as indicated, and reacts one hour in bed.

34. POULTICES

Use and Abuse of Poultices

There are eight conditions for which poultices should be employed: (1) to relieve pain and congestion and to act as a counterirritant; (2) to reduce inflammation; (3) to promote absorption, favor resolution, or hasten the formation of a head in abscesses; (4) to diminish tissue swelling and tension; (5) to soften crusted lesions; (6) to encourage muscle relaxation; (7) to stimulate healthy granulation; and (8) to perform the office of a deodorant and in a sense an antiseptic or disinfectant.

Certain medications used in a poultice, as in the mustard plaster, can lead to blistering or ulceration. A poultice applied after pus develops is sometimes a detriment, as the poultice may encourage the growth of bacteria. If pus increases, discontinue poultices. The heat retaining capacity of the material used is more important than the material itself. In pneumonia, peritonitis, and other deep-seated inflammations, the poultice should be large enough to cover a surface area equal to the size of the organ being treated. It should be covered with plastic, and should be removed if it becomes cold. A charcoal poultice is both deodorant and antiseptic. A layer of powdered charcoal may be sprinkled on the surface of infected wounds or ulcers.

Clay and Glycerine Poultice

Use fine quality clay obtained from several inches below the surface of the earth, containing no rocks or coarse grains. Put it through a fine hardware cloth if necessary, and sterilize in the oven at 350° for sufficient length of time to thoroughly heat all portions. Reconstitute to the moisture content of clay as it ordinarily appears in soil, and then moisten with several tablespoons of glycerin. Use the clay and glycerin as a poultice.

To reclaim the clay, pour water over the clay and allow it to settle, pouring off the fluid that collects on top, and again sterilizing it in the oven. With this process some of the beneficial factors are lost from the clay and it can be used only once.

Clay Dressings

Take a good grade of fine clay, make a paste with water, and apply directly to the skin surface in cases of skin rashes and other skin diseases. Cover with several layers of cotton cloth or gauze. Keep the poultice moist for 6-10 hours by frequent applications of water. Rinse thoroughly, dry, and allow an hour or two to elapse before reapplying the moist dressing. Clay holds water well and has a therapeutic benefit in most inflammatory skin diseases.[96]

Flaxseed Poultice

Flaxseed can be purchased from a health food store or supermarket. It is often used for cooking, for constipation, to make gels, and it has a medicated quality that makes it useful in therapeutics. One tablespoon of flaxseed ground in a seed mill or blender and mixed with one cup of water brought to a boil, will make enough paste for a poultice large enough to cover the front of the abdomen. Take a paper towel and spread the material completely over the towel. It may be laid directly on the skin of the affected area. Cover completely with a plastic, allowing the plastic to extend over the edges an inch on all sides. Hold the poultice in place with a roller bandage, an ace bandage, or a 50 to 60″ strip of cloth specially prepared for this purpose, cutting a strip from a bedsheet or other long piece, wrapping it around the entire body or an extremity and pinning it in place. Make a neat, snug bandage. Leave the poultice on from 30 minutes to 8 hours. At the end of the time, remove the poultice, sponge the surface clean with a damp washcloth, and friction the area of the poultice with an alcohol sponge, or a cold mitten friction. Dry thoroughly and replace clothing.

Hops Poultice

The fresh leaves, or dry leaves moistened with hot water, may be whizzed in a blender with a little water and spread out on folded paper towel or facial tissue to make a poultice of the proper size to cover the affected area. Proceed as with the flaxseed poultice above.

Comfrey and Smartweed Poultice

As with hops, the fresh leaves of comfrey and smartweed may be used. The dried leaves may be substituted, if necessary. Simply moisten the dried leaves with water and proceed as before. For the fresh leaves, proceed as described above for hops.

Mustard Plaster

Place a large platter or metal tray where it can get warm, not hot. Stir dry mustard and ordinary wheat flour together as follows: 1 tablespoon of mustard to 4 tablespoons of flour for an adult; 1 tablespoon of mustard to 8 tablespoons of flour for a child; and 1 tablespoon of mustard to 12 tablespoons of flour for an infant. Add enough tepid water to make a paste thin enough to spread, but not so thin as to run. Place a cloth (an old handkerchief is best) on the warm platter, spreading the paste from the center toward the edges, leaving a margin wide enough to lap over well on all sides. Do not remove the poultice from the warm platter until the patient is ready for the application. One thin layer of cotton cloth should separate the mustard paste from the patient's skin. After the poultice has been put in place, cover with a large piece of plastic to protect the patient's clothing. Over that place a towel, folded or flat, which can be pinned to hold the mustard plaster in place. At this point, if a greater reaction is desired, a stupe can be made by simply applying a single moderately hot fomentation for the duration of the plaster. Leave the plaster on 20 minutes. If the patient complains of stinging and burning, or if the skin becomes well reddened before the time is up, the plaster should be removed. Wipe the area well with cotton or tissue dipped in mineral oil or cooking oil to remove all mustard traces. Cover the areas well with warm flannel or terrycloth towel. Pin it in place to a snug-fitting sweater or cotton shirt. Leave on overnight.[104] Use for pain in arthritic joints, for backache, and to improve the circulation.[105]

35. SINUS PACK

Equipment

1. Two trays of ice cubes
2. Two small dry towels
3. Hot fomentation for the spine
4. Set of 3 fomentations alternating with cold to the chest
5. Hot foot bath

Procedure

1. Proceed first with a set of three fomentations to the chest, 3 minutes hot and 30 seconds cold. Leave the third hot fomentation on the chest throughout the remainder of the treatment.
2. Put one tray of ice cubes in a small dry towel. Fold it over to make a pack 5 x 10″. Make a second pack.
3. Put one end of the treatment table or bed against the wall.
4. Put one ice pack under the back of the neck centered on the edge of the cranium.
5. Wet the top of the head slightly with water and place the second ice pack on the top of the head. Hold the pack in place with a pillow.
6. Fold a small towel lengthwise, grasp it in the center edge with one hand, and fold down the ends 90° from the central point as shown in the illustration.

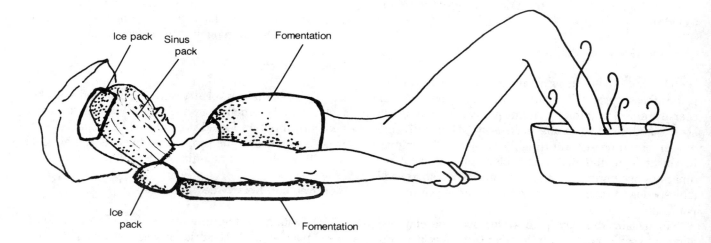

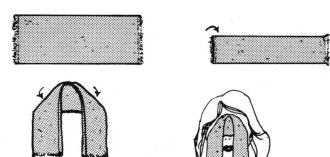

Place it on the face for protection, leaving the nose exposed through the slit.

7. Use a single fomentation, folded as the towel is folded. Place it over the towel on the face. Leave on exactly three minutes! This is a stimulating treatment. Remove the fomentation and towel.

8. Wring another small towel from ice water and drape it on the face, molding it to the skin over the red area. There should be no delay between removal of the hot fomentation and replacement by the cold compress. Leave on thirty seconds! After drying briskly, repeat steps 6, 7, and 8 three times. Finish off with a cold mitten friction, beginning with the face, or use a contrast shower.

36. THE EYE COMPRESS

Hot or cold compresses to the eye may be made easily by putting some cotton in the bowl of a long-handled wooden spoon, wrapping it with gauze or cotton, and tying in place (see illustration). Dip into hot water.

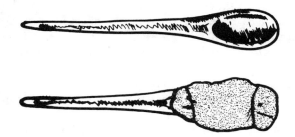

The excess water can be expressed between the layers of a folded towel, and the compress applied to the eye. For such conditions as acute glaucoma and acute iridocyclitis the compress should be used faithfully for 20 minutes every hour; for sties it may be used 20 minutes every three to four hours until the sty points and opens, or subsides. In the acute diseases mentioned above, use the treatments as first aid while arranging for the services of an eye specialist, and continue the treatments as long as the pain

persists or the condition of the eye demands. Heat is beneficial in any condition of the anterior segment of the eyeball. Cold allays pain and promotes healing by relieving congestion.[106]

37. DAILY COOL BATH

In the winter, the routine use of the cool bath trains the skin to react promptly, and thus reduces the danger of taking cold or sensing an unpleasant reaction as a result of a momentary or accidental chilling. The importance of the daily cool bath is far greater than is generally understood. It stimulates the thyroid to normal activity. It keeps the bone marrow functioning properly. It is an important prophylaxis against colds. The young should be trained to take a cool or cold bath daily. The physical development will be encouraged. Even the morals may be strengthened by the discipline required and the good accomplished. General vigor and muscle tone will be increased.

38. SHOWER BATH OR RAIN BATH

Indications

1. Same as for short cold bath
2. Stimulation in prolonged obstetrical labor
3. Acclimatization in extreme sensitivity to cold
4. Strengthens against taking colds or influenza

Equipment

1. Shower cap
2. Coarse washcloth, luffa sponge, or stiff bath brush
3. Hot foot bath

Procedure

1. Prepare a hot foot bath for all neutral or cool showers. If tub and shower are together, hot water at about 110° may be put in the bathtub about 2 inches deep. See precautions under hot foot baths.
2. Adjust the water temperature to the proper level for the treatment desired: hot, warm, tepid, cool or cold.
3. The force of the spray should be at as high a pressure as can be obtained—especially is this true for cold showers which are far more readily tolerated if the pressure is high than if there is a gentle, fine spray.
4. The patient must step quickly into the hot foot bath and then plunge directly into the shower, beginning at once to rub the skin briskly with the luffa, brush, or coarse washcloth at the very point where the shower strikes the skin. As the friction accompanies

the cold or warm water, a more pronounced reaction will occur.

5. Continue the bath different lengths of time for various temperatures: hot, 2 to 10 minutes; warm and tepid, 2 to 10 minutes; cool, 1 to 5 minutes; and cold, 30 to 180 seconds.

6. A "graduated shower" can be obtained by starting with a warm shower and gradually reducing the temperature to cold. Many persons find this procedure more pleasant than stepping directly into a cold shower.

7. An alternating hot and cold shower can be used as a mini-treatment or as a finish for fomentations or fever treatments.

8. When the shower is finished, the person should friction dry with a coarse towel, rubbing the skin until it glows red.

9. When the shower is used as a treatment for disease, a reaction time of about 30 minutes should be spent in bed; however, the shower may be used as a daily hygienic measure and can precede or follow the routine physical or mental activities.

39. FULL BODY PACK (BLANKET PACK) FOR FEVER TREATMENT

Indications

1. Relieves pain and tension
2. Elevates body temperature to mild or high fever
3. Mobilizes white blood cells in the bloodstream
4. Stimulates production of antibodies
5. Sweats out many body wastes and disease toxins
6. Flushes the glands and organs

Contraindications

1. Advanced age or debilitated condition
2. Grave physical defects or illness
3. History of heat stroke or hyperpyrexia

Procedure

1. Make sure of a recent good bowel movement even if an enema is required.
2. Lay 3 blankets on the bed, the top one extending well up over the head, to be used as a hood.
3. Cover the top blanket with a plastic sheet, then put down a set of heavy fomentations—three or four may be needed to extend from the patient's neck to his thighs. Cover well with three to five thicknesses of towels. An electric blanket turned high may be substituted for the steam packs if preferred.

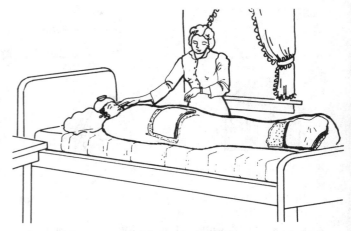

Blanket Pack. One side of the pack is left open to show the layers, towels, fomentations, plastic sheeting, and blankets. An ice bag is at the patient's head and the nurse is taking the pulse at the temple.

4. The patient, wrapped in a sheet with a towel around the neck, lies on the fomentations which are then tucked up along both sides.

5. Next, a fomentation is laid over the abdomen, and another wrapped around the feet. Check to make certain the skin is not overheating.

6. Cover the patient with the plastic sheet, then the top blanket, well tucked in to hold the packs close. This blanket is brought over the head as a hood, leaving the face out. The second and third blanket may be used as needed.

7. Take the temperature and pulse every 15 minutes.

8. The patient remains in the pack from 45 minutes to several hours, determined by the level of the temperature required. The mouth temperature may be held at 102° by loosening the blankets, or may be taken up to 104° if needed. When the oral temperature is over 103°, take readings of both pulse and temperature every five minutes. If the pulse approaches 160, or the temperature goes over 105°, terminate the treatment. (See also Fever Treatments in an earlier section.)

9. Sweating should be profuse. If the treatment lasts over an hour or the temperature goes over 102°, uncover the head and keep the face sponged with cool cloths. Place a cold compress on the forehead.

10. Give a minimum of one pint of saline per hour when the temperature is over 102°. Patients who take a sufficient amount of fluids tolerate a long treatment much better than those who do not take fluids well. Offer water every 5-10 minutes.

11. Remove the patient from the pack and finish with a shower or sponge bath.[107]

40. LOWER HALF BODY PACK

The lower half body pack consists of two heavy double fomentations placed across a bed or massage table. Pad and cover the fomentations with towels in such a manner that when the patient is placed on the pack, it extends from the mid-shoulder blades to the lower edge of the hips. For comfort, elevate the head and flex the knees over a bolster. Cover with a sheet, then with one to three blankets tucked in well. The patient remains in the pack for 45 minutes. Finish the treatment with a cold mitten friction or a cool shower.

41. HOT HIP AND LEG PACK

According to Abbott[106] this treatment is one of the most efficient derivative measures in hydrotherapy. When used with an ice bag to the congested part, it is more effective.

This pack includes the feet, legs, thighs, and hips to the waist. A hot water bottle should be placed at the feet and a second between the legs or behind the thighs. The general procedure is identical to the heating trunk pack.

42. FLUID ADMINISTRATION

General Aspects

Fluid admistration is essential in illness to avoid dehydration, or to correct it once it has developed.

Signs of dehydration include fainting, dizziness, chapped lips, dry mouth and skin, cough, nausea, increased temperature, fast pulse, low blood pressure, and higher than usual readings from the laboratory on such chemistries as hemoglobin, cholesterol, blood urea nitrogen (BUN), sodium, etc.

Of course, the primary method of administration of fluids is by mouth. If the patient is able to take oral fluids, this is the safest, cheapest, most convenient and comfortable method, and by all means should be used. The next simplest and safest method is the retention enema. It should receive second choice as a mode of administration of fluids since intravenous fluids are expensive, require special setup for administration, and specially trained personnel for the venepuncture, to say nothing of the fact that administration of IV fluids is not without some hazard to the health of the patient.

With any heating treatment that elevates the body temperature, one to two glasses of water should be given before the treatment, and should be offered constantly during the treatment. When the oral temperature reaches 101° to 102°, the fluid intake should be about two cups per hour minimum, unless the patient is not sweating. If sweating is copious, much chloride will be lost in the sweat and should be replaced by the use of saline (1 teaspoon of salt to two cups of water) instead of plain water, unless the patient is being treated for high blood pressure, in which case the loss of salt may be desirable.

Use about two quarts of water per 24 hours if there is no evidence of excessive loss of fluids from diarrhea, vomiting, or sweating. If there is fever, or if heating treatments are given, more fluid will be needed. If there is much sputum production or saliva lost, tears produced or weeping skin lesions, correspondingly more fluid will be required to keep the person well hydrated.

The Retention Enema

The retention enema method of administration of fluids when oral administration is not possible is the mainstay of fluid balance in a home situation. Minerals lost by vomiting, diarrhea, or sweating can also be replaced by retention enema if necessary. A solution can be prepared by the following recipe: simmer two tablespoons of wheat bran in two cups of water for 5-10 minutes. Strain and add 2 teaspoons of salt. Add sufficient water to the mixture to make two quarts (8 cups). If the patient has not eaten for a day or two, it may be desirable to add 2-3 tablespoons of white table sugar to the mixture for its protein-sparing effect. Use the administration procedure described in the section on enemas.

Precaution should be taken to avoid overloading any patient with fluids. Those with nephritis or congestive heart failure can be overloaded with both salt and water. Babies and children can be overloaded with water and develop water intoxication, a serious condition of dilute blood that can be fatal. A typical history is that the parents believe an enema will cure some malady, and give three or four enemas within a few minutes or hours. It is especially likely to overload the child if very little of the enema fluid is returned. Both adults and children can get pulmonary edema from too much fluid. The danger, however is *much greater* with intravenous fluids than with enemas or oral fluids. In addition, phlebitis at the injection site and pyrogenic reactions (fever) from intravenous fluid administration do occasionally occur, and it cannot be considered an innocuous procedure to give IV fluids.

Intravenous Fluids

Interestingly, the use of coconut water for IV fluids has been considered a cheap and readily available source of fluid containing the requisite electrolytes. We have not used this method ourselves, but it is described by Dr.

Quazi M. Iqbal of the Department of Orthopedic Surgery at the University of Kebangssan in Malaysia. We describe it for its interest to those who have the conviction that in nature is provided a simple remedy for every malady of man. Dr. Iqbal infused the coconut water directly from the fruit into the vein of the patient without any prior treatment of the water in 15 surgical cases. Only a single infusion of 600 ml into the antecubital vein was used in each case.

Young green coconuts of five to six months were chosen as are commonly available commercially. Fruits were inspected for cracks. Strips of husk were raised on either side as by the local vendor, and tied in a knot; the loop was used for suspension. The surface of the coconut was sterilized and the husk sliced until the resilient inner shell was exposed. With a large gauge needle the preliminary puncture was made and some of the fluid captured and inspected. The first needle was then withdrawn, the infusion needle inserted in its place, and the infusion commenced.[102] It would seem wise that the tubing be carefully inspected for particulate matter, although persons acquainted with the method believe the likelihood of particles entering the needle to be very low.

Subcutaneous Fluids

In small babies, children, and others who cannot take fluids by mouth, rectum, or IV, the subcutaneous administration may be life-saving. A syringe should be filled with the proper quantity of sterilized, pyrogen-free fluid. The skin of the back or outer aspect of the thighs is a good site for injection. A baby can be given 25 to 50 cc. in these locations and an adult 200 to 300 cc. by push-in. The subcutaneous tissue will be noted to swell with the fluid. The injection may be repeated in the same site as often as needed.

43. IRRIGATIONS (NASAL, MOUTH, PHARYNX, TONSILLAR, EAR)

The treatment is excellent for cleansing surfaces, for delivering heat and for giving a massaging or friction treatment. It can substitute for a gargle or the usual mouthwash if the area is too tender for other treatments.

Equipment and Materials

1. Use a hand-held bulb syringe, four to ten ounce size, or a pulsating dental irrigator, such as a Water Pik.
2. Use hot water (110°) or saline for nasal irrigation.
3. For streptococcal infections, use one quart of water into which one clove of garlic has been blended. If a Water Pik is used, the tip of the irrigator can be cut

off to give a larger stream under less pressure. Use one of the lowest pressure settings. Strain the solution through a nylon stocking or gauze if particles clog the tubing. The solution may be used hot or cold. Charcoal is also useful for bacterial sore throats such as streptococcal or diphtherial. Mix 1-4 tablespoons per quart of warm or hot water. The bacteria adhere to charcoal. Garlic inhibits growth of bacteria, fungi and viruses.

Indications

1. Hay fever
2. Colds
3. Aphthous ulcers of the mouth or pharynx
4. Acute tonsillitis or peritonsillar abscess
5. Streptococcal or diphtherial sore throats
6. Asthma

Procedure

This irrigation may be self-administered. Fill the syringe with hot water or saline, expelling all air and completely filling the syringe. Bend over a sink or basin, or administer in bed with a basin held to catch the run-off water. For a peritonsillar abscess, direct the spray toward the back of the throat, using as much heat and pressure as can be tolerated to massage the tissues and encourage dissipation of the infection. Allow the run-off to escape into the sink or basin. Use one quart or more of hot water or irrigation solution.

For a nasal irrigation, insert the syringe nozzle into the nose and hold the nostril closed around the nozzle with a finger. The nostril can be completely occluded by wrapping the end of the nozzle with a large rubber band just bulky enough that it wedges snugly inside the nose

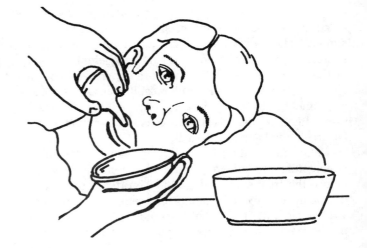

upon insertion. Squeeze the bulb of the syringe with a steady stream, allowing the run-off to escape through the opposite nostril into the sink.

The irrigation is an excellent treatment for a beginning cold when used at 110° to 115° for about 30 minutes. It is said by some never to fail to prevent the cold from developing if it is used within the first 24 hours. A peritonsillar abscess, acute pharyngitis, or tonsillitis will respond miraculously to this simple remedy if begun early. Be persistent in treatment of the more serious sore throats for a few days after symptoms subside. We treated a young lady who had a peritonsillar abscess with such severe swelling on one side that she could speak only with the voice directed through the nose as in cleft palate, could not swallow, and found it very difficult even to open her mouth. She experienced intense pain in the ear of the affected side. She could not eat, or swallow her own saliva.

Within three days of beginning hot saline irrigations to the nose and pharynx, hot baths, fomentations over the throat and ear, and charcoal poultices, her speech was normal and fluids could be swallowed. She was entirely well after 4 days of intensive treatment.

44. IRRIGATIONS OF THE EAR

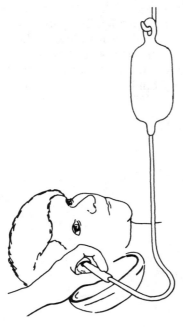

Use an irrigation setup similar to an enema bag with a small rubber or glass tube with rounded edges, or one may use an ordinary bulb syringe. Use water from 99° to 101°. Use little pressure. A tray or bowl should be held firmly against the cheek and neck below the ear. The operator should pull the ear upward and backward to straighten the canal and direct the stream of water forward and downward. An ear syringe should be pressed steadily to deliver water at a constant rate under very gentle pressure. If the water is hot the patient may experience some currents of fluid movement in the nearby semi-circular canals, causing sensations of faintness, dizziness or nausea.

Irrigation of the ear is used in acute inflammation of the ear, to remove hardened wax, to remove insects or foreign bodies, and in eczema of the ear canal. Ear wax may be softened by dropping a few drops of plain water or a little warm olive oil into the canal. Allow the fluid or oil to remain at least one-half hour before tipping the head upright again. Repeat three or four times at daily intervals, and then irrigate the ear.

45. MEDICATED BATHS

Alkaline Baths (Soda Baths)

To a full tub of water, approximately 20-30 gallons, at 94° to 98°, add about one cup of baking soda or commercial grade sodium bicarbonate. The patient should sit in the tub, and with a cup, dip the alkaline water onto the knees, shoulders, and abdomen, so that the water continually bathes all portions of the skin. Baking soda has a slightly anesthetic property; this treatment is good for drug reactions, poison ivy, itching, eczema, hives, bee stings, ant stings, heat rash, sensitivities to plants or chemicals, sunburns, and other general skin reactions.

The patient may stay in the bath for 30 minutes to an hour if necessary. When the time is up, the patient should stand in the tub for a few seconds to allow the excess water to drip from the skin. The skin should be patted dry, or the patient allowed to sit on the edge of the tub or on a stool until the skin is entirely dry. A heater or electric fan may hasten the drying process.

Starch Bath

Stir approximately one cup of dry starch into a shallow tub of water at about 94° to 98°. The patient should sit in the water for about 20 to 30 minutes, or longer if necessary. A cup may be used to dip the water onto all skin surfaces that are affected. Stir the water to keep the starch suspended. The bath is given for skin irritations, about the same as the alkaline bath. Finish the bath in the same way, allowing the patient to dry in air by patting, fanning or dripping. For diaper rash the water need not be discarded after one use but may be used repeatedly.

Oatmeal Bath

One pound of uncooked oatmeal is tied loosely in a large piece of gauze and hung or held under the bathtub spigot in such a way that the water runs through the oatmeal, using the hot water first to soften the oatmeal and encourage the elution of the starch. After the tub has been filled, the bag of oatmeal is left in the bath water, and the patient may use the bag to sponge the surface of the body. One heaping cup of uncooked rolled oats, ground fine in a blender, can be substituted for the one pound bag. It is stirred into the bathtub, or used in a whirlpool as it will not affect the agitator. The patient should remain in the tub for 20 to 30 minutes or longer and finish by patting dry according to the method given for the alkaline bath. Use for poison ivy, eczema, hives, and any itching affliction.[110]

Oxygen Bath (Peroxide Bath)

Indications

1. Any condition requiring a powerful stimulation to the skin circulation
2. Insomnia or nervousness
3. Asthma
4. High blood pressure
5. Pemphigus
6. Diabetic gangrene
7. Dermatitis

Procedure

1. Fill the bath tub with approximately 30 gallons of water at 98° to 100°.
2. Dissolve 1 tablespoon of potassium permanganate in 1 quart of boiling water and pour it into the bath.
3. Stir in 1½ tablespoons of sulfuric acid.
4. Add 13-16 ounces of hydrogen peroxide; effervescence begins at once. If preferred, a more expensive but sometimes more readily available material may be used to produce the oxygen bubbles in the water. Dissolve 300 grams of sodium perborate ($NaBO_3$) by sprinkling uniformly into the bath water. Next sprinkle on the catalyzer, 1 tablespoon of manganese borate ($Mn_3(BO_3)_2$). The bubbles begin in 1-2 minutes and continue for 15-20 minutes.
5. Maintain the water temperature at 98° to 100°. The patient should sit still in the bath. The sensation of mild prickling should be pleasant and agreeable.
6. After about 20 minutes the patient arises from the tub, gently blots the skin dry, dresses slowly and retires to bed to sleep.

Sulfur Bath

Use about one-third to one-half the usual quantity of water for a bath; about 10-15 gallons is used for this bath. Stir one-half to one ounce of potassium sulfate in the 10 to 15 gallons of water at 102°. The patient sits in the water and dips the medicated water onto the skin surface for 30 to 60 minutes. This bath is used for acne, lice, impetigo, infected eczema, and other skin diseases. Following the bath, the skin should be blotted dry without friction.

CHAPTER TWELVE

Special Classes of Treatments

Stimulants and the Tonics

Stimulant and tonic treatments are given in cases where the body is performing below par. These treatments call forth energy not being tapped by the usual vegetative and nutritive processes of the body. They are useful in convalesence from acute illness, in many chronic illnesses, in anemia, hypothyroidism, constipation, somnolence and conversely some cases of insomnia, obesity, diabetes, and muscular weakness or paralysis.

A list of tonic measures includes cold mitten friction, salt glow, pail pour, cold douche, wet sheet pack, dripping sheet rub, and cold shower or bath.

Sedatives

Use sedatives for those who have hyperthyroidism, insomnia, hyperactivity, nervousness, mental illness, rigidity, and spasticity, chorea, and epilepsy.

Other indications for sedatives include pain, both deep and superficial, peptic ulcers, hemorrhoids, dysmenorrhea, colic, burns, sprains, bruises and fractures, pruritis (itching), hives and heat rashes, numbness and tingling, burning and smarting.

The sedative treatments include the neutral or warm bath, a wet sheet pack starting with a neutral temperature, prolonged mild hot baths, heating compresses, prolonged mild fomentations or mild hot foot baths with cool compresses to the head, heating pad set at the lowest setting or a hot water bottle to the abdomen or back, and gentle stroking massage.

Natural Expectorants (Cough Syrups)

Natural expectorants are capable of causing watery bronchial secretions to increase in order that thick or mucoid materials or products of inflammation may be removed with greater ease. Water is the best natural ex-pectorant, and should be consumed in copious quantities. Garlic acts as an expectorant since the active ingredient of garlic is eliminated through the lungs; this causes the lungs to give off a more watery secretion, enabling the person to more readily expectorate thick bronchial plugs or dry, heavy mucus.

Hot compresses applied to the chest will also increase the ability to bring up thick secretions from the lungs. A fever treatment or Russian steam bath is very efficient in assisting with the expectoration. Expectorants are useful in asthma, chronic bronchitis, pneumonia, diphtheria, whooping cough, and other pulmonary problems.

Diuretics

Any agent that increases the production and flow of urine is spoken of as a diuretic. The drug diuretics act by overtaxing or poisoning the kidneys in one way or another, forcing the flow of fluid from the blood stream to increase the output of urine.

There are four different pharmacologic actions of drug medications producing diuresis:

1. *An increase in arterial pressure:* At any time the blood pressure increases within the kidney, more fluid is forced out of the renal capillaries and into the urine collecting ducts, resulting in greater urine output. *Examples:* norepinephrine type drugs which increase arterial pressure, and digitalis types which increase cardiac output. Both of these categories of drugs are toxic.

2. *Drug effect on the kidney tubules to interfere with the reabsorption of water or other substances:* Examples: The mercurial diuretics pharmacologically interfere with the reabsorption of sodium and chloride into the blood stream which causes water to be retained in the kidney tubules. Potassium is increased or decreased depending on whether the initial

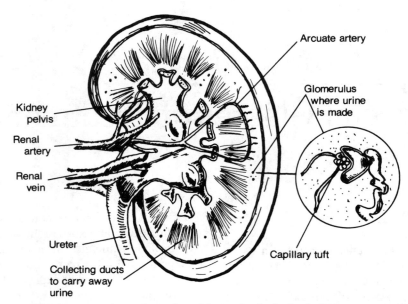

The kidney is in many ways the most marvelous piece of equipment in the body. It inspects every drop of blood repeatedly. As much as 20% of the output of blood from the heart can go to the kidneys for evaluation, adjustment, and purification. The small insert is the functioning unit, the glomerulus. The tiny capillary tuft is the filter, holding back the blood cells, but pushing out the plasma through holes in the capillary. The cup-shaped apparatus receives the plasma and adjusts and purifies it and returns most of it to the blood stream, keeping out only the wastes and a very small amount of water, which it sends on down the tubes to the bladder for elimination.

secretory rate is low or high. The thiazides cause an increased excretion of sodium and chloride which accomplishes the same type of water retention in the tubule, increasing the flow of urine. Both of these categories of drugs are toxic.

3. *An increase in the solid materials in the urine:* Accumulation of solids in the kidney tubules causes an increase in the water needed to keep the solids in solution. With the increase in solids in the urine comes an increase in osmotic pressure within the collecting tubules. *Examples:* Substances such as mannitol and urea when present in the blood stream are filtered from the capillaries in the kidney into the tubules which attract the fluid from the blood because of the increase in the osmotic pressure within the tubules. Water is not reabsorbed from the tubule, and passes out as urine. The elevated blood glucose in the uncontrolled diabetic, when exceeding the renal threshold, spills over into the urine and produces a similar osmotic diuresis.

4. *Selective dilatation of arterioles within the kidney to increase filtration.* Example: Such substances as caffeine dilate the arterioles that go to the tiny tubules that collect the expressed

fluid. These substances act through the nerves causing a tax on the nerves in many parts of the body. The dilated arterioles permit a larger volume of blood to flow into the structure that makes the urine, therefore increasing the fluid within the collecting ducts.

When fluid accumulates, as in advanced hepatitis or nephritis, sweating baths and packs may be helpful. In ordinary conditions of fluid retention, measures that are even more simple may be all that is required: getting plenty of sleep at night and perhaps a nap in the daytime, elevating the feet to promote the return of lymph fluid to the blood stream, and the wearing of elastic stockings or ace bandages on the lower extremities to encourage resorption of fluid that would otherwise pool in the legs. Cold baths act as a diuretic by constricting the peripheral circulation and increasing the intrarenal pressure.[111]

Other treatments having a diuretic effect include the full hot blanket pack, electric light bath, Russian bath, hot tub bath, and alternating hot and cold applications with friction to the lower sternum and lumbar spine, heating trunk pack, fomentations to the lumbar spine, as well as copious water drinking, and the restriction of sugar, salt, and oils in the diet. The diuretic teas include buchu, burdock, cornsilk, watermelon seed, golden seal, and comfrey. These all have a nutritive effect on the kidneys more like the action of item four above. Horsetail grass is diuretic, but may have toxic properties, and need not be used.

Treatments to bring about diuresis are especially beneficial in acute or chronic nephritis, uremia, cystitis, eclampsia, food poisoning, and other types of poisoning in which the kidneys are involved. In order to avoid water overload, remember to measure carefully the total fluid intake when the kidneys have failed, as they cannot adjust the fluid level well in the blood.

Gastrointestinal Stimulants

All factors to increase the function of the digestive organs are classed as stimulants. Treatments that will increase the muscular or secretory activity of the digestive organs are included here:

1. Hot or heating trunk pack
2. Fomentations to the abdomen
3. Moist abdominal bandage
4. Alternating hot and cold compresses to the spine, abdomen and liver
5. Hot water bottle or heating pad over the abdomen after meals. (Heat on the abdomen before meals acts as a sedative.)
6. Ice bag, cold water drinking, or cold compress over the stomach before meals

These treatments are useful in all forms of indigestion and chronic congestion of the digestive organs, in low hydrochloric acid production, pernicious anemia, hiatus hernia, and dyspepsia from any cause.

CHAPTER THIRTEEN

Diseases and Their Home Remedies

Abscess

Application of heat to an abscess in a closed space is often contraindicated. The application of heat to an infection tends to draw the infection to a central point, an undesirable process in a closed space. An example is that of the appendix. If an acute appendicitis is caused to "collect" in the appendix, the appendix may swell and rupture. Similarly, an abscess in a tooth should be scattered rather than collected. Usually the application of heat in these cases will cause an increase in the discomfort that the patient is suffering, whereas applying cold relieves it.

In all abscesses, as well as appendicitis and tooth infection, if the treatments are begun early enough the inflammation will clear and the abscess will not form. Of course, this is the most desirable course, as an abscess is always associated with more or less tissue destruction, followed by scarring. Both charcoal and garlic poultices may be applied with good results.

Appendicitis

While the treatment of choice for acute appendicitis is surgical removal of the appendix, there are several things that may be done to relieve pain, discomfort and fever while the diagnosis is being established, or the most favorable time for surgery is being sought. A hot foot bath will help to relieve congestion in the appendix. In the early stages there is a possibility that with prompt and vigorous treatment the inflammation will subside and the appendix heal itself. That this often occurs is attested to by the many appendices seen by the pathologist and diagnosed as "fibrotic appendix"—a scar has developed at some time in the past due to appendicitis. It may be desirable to use a hot hip and leg pack with an ice bag over the appendix.

The physiologic action of the ice bag or the hot water bottle is about the same. Both cause redness of the skin, but either heat or cold is, to a certain extent, dissipated by the blood stream and does not penetrate far beneath the surface. For most people there is more relief of pain in acute appendicitis from the use of the ice bag than from a hot water bottle. Use the ice bag an hour on and fifteen minutes off. During these 15 minutes hot fomentations may be used to good advantage.[105] Charcoal as a poultice, with hops or smartweed, is effective both to relieve pain and to dispel inflammation.

Arthritis

1. Osteoarthritis and general joint pain

A method for giving hydrotherapy using a heating pad to apply heat to a joint is as follows: Wring out a large towel from tap water, and wrap it around the affected joint. Cover the towel completely with two layers of plastic wrap. A large plastic bag can be used, and for an extremity, both ends of the bag can be opened and the bag used as a sleeve over the wet towel, the excess being folded over and taped with scotch or masking tape. Next, place a heating pad over the plastic cover and attach in place, turning the control to low or medium. Apply this once a day for one to two hours at a time. A radio placed at the bedside, using the same electrical outlet as the heating pad, will crackle with static as a warning if the heating pad is getting wet and beginning to short. Tune the radio to a blank place on the dial and set the volume loud enough to attract attention.

2. Rheumatoid arthritis

Contrast baths have been used for rheumatoid arthritis with considerable relief. The temperatures recommended have been 50° to 65° (10° to 18° C.) for cold water and 99° to 110° (37.8° to 43.3° C.) for the hot. Alternation in the temperature is considered an activator of the peripheral reflexes to increase circulation to the joint.

For advanced and crippling arthritis, the continuous or hammock bath rigged with clamps in constantly flowing water offers much relief. The water should be about 98°, and the room somewhat warm. Continue the bath for 2 hours, five or six days a week. It is remarkable how quickly patients feel relief. Usually they are enabled to stop their medications after the second or third bath. One patient walked again after the tenth bath, which he had been unable to do for three years.[106]

3. Gout

An elevation of uric acid in the blood results in crystals of uric acid which deposit in the tissues around joints and in the soft tissues of skin and kidneys as well as elsewhere. For those with certain kidney diseases or an hereditary predisposition, a diet high in purines often produces gout. Purines, which are high in most foods of animal origin and low in most foods from plant sources, are broken down into uric acid. Yeasts of all kinds (baker's, brewer's, and food yeasts) all promote a high uric acid in the blood. Large doses of charcoal by mouth—ten tablets four times a day for ten days—charcoal baths and compresses promote a fall in the blood uric acid. Mud baths have also been suggested as useful in gout.

4. Infectious Arthritis

About one-third of patients with chronic infectious arthritis derive substantial benefits from fever treatments, one-third derive only moderate benefit, and one-third little or no help. In gonococcal arthritis, swelling and pain is often astonishingly helped. Patients suffering from hypertrophic arthritis (osteoarthritis) receive temporary benefit, and the fever treatments may be used along with general arthritis treatment of diet and physical conditioning.

Asthma

One spinal pack will do much to abort or relieve an attack of asthma. Make up a heavy double steam pack, lay it on a plastic sheet on the bed and cover it with a towel. The person lies on it so that the pack comes up to the neck. Cover the person warmly in winter and lightly in summer, using a light fan directed to the face for comfort. The patient should lie quietly for 30 minutes. Finish the treatment with a sponge bath or an alcohol rub and coarse towel friction rubdown.

Anything that increases perspiration of the skin will encourage increased activity of the mucous membranes. Since secretions become thickened and rubbery in asthma, the increased activity loosens secretions and promotes expectoration and clearing of the bronchial tree. Asthma may be relieved by the Russian bath, but will return with redoubled force if there is any inadvertent draft exposure following the bath. To prevent asthma, give fever treatments one to three times weekly while the patient is not in a severe attack.

Back Pain, Low

Place the patient in a lower-half body pack for 20 to 25 minutes to relax all the tendons and ligaments of the lower back. Remove the pack and turn the patient on the right side. Place the right leg straight down and flex the left knee up as far as it will go, with the toes hooked over the back of the right knee if possible. Pull the hip forward, and push the shoulder backward (elbow out of the way) to achieve a torsion position of the trunk. Simultaneously push the shoulder back and pull the hip forward, allowing the left knee to slide off the table and point downward toward the floor. Using some force, slightly hyperextend the joints involved. Make the manipulation firm, but gentle. There need not be any cracking sound. The objective is to mobilize the joints and increase the circulation to the area.

Next, turn the patient on his left side, left leg down and right knee drawn up, right shoulder slanted backward and right hip forward. With the same simultaneous motion as before, push the shoulder back and pull the hip forward, knee sliding off the table. This action mobilizes the sacroiliac junction and increases the circulation to the joint. Sometimes a faint snapping sound occurs because of motion in the tendons, not actually involving the bones. Finish with a shower or a sponge bath. The patient should allow 30 minutes reaction time in bed.

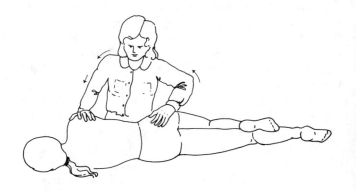

Blood Pressure

In general, it has been found that hot baths lower blood pressure and cold baths raise it. Steam baths and sweating have a salutary effect on hypertension, with a drop in both systolic and diastolic pressures.[114] Strasburger found that the results from the use of heat and cold are complicated, and that a cold bath may produce an initial rise in blood pressure, followed by a fall and again by a second rise. He noticed, also, that hot baths above 104° (40° C.) often gave a blood pressure above normal. While warm baths are generally associated with a fall of pressure, a neutral bath at 93° to 95° (34° to 35° C.) produced no change in blood pressure.[115]

Other measures also should be taken to combat an elevated blood pressure, chief of which are salt and oil restriction. The average adult needs only about 100 to 750 milligrams of salt. This means about one-tenth teaspoon of salt per day. Most Americans get from six to forty times this amount.[116] The food alone contains sufficient salt to supply all the body needs even if no salt is added in preparation. In order to reduce the diet to a 500 milligram salt intake, dieticians need to struggle to remove many foods that are naturally high in sodium or salt. All dairy products are naturally high in salt, as are many meats. Many processed foods are high in added salt, and such products as beef or chicken bouillon cubes may be 50% or more salt. All canned vegetables and most baby foods, unless specifically stated on the label, have considerable quantities of salt in them. In susceptible individuals, a high salt diet produces a gradual rise in blood pressure from childhood to old age. Children of susceptible parents generally tend to develop cravings for salt. If the craving develops, the child is creating an increased risk for middle age hypertension with the complications of stroke, kidney disease, and arteriosclerosis which accompany high blood pressure.

Bronchitis and Coughs

Spread a plastic on the bed and place on it two double steam packs crosswise over the area where the patient will lie, from neck to waistline. Cover well with towels and have the patient lie down. For comfort, elevate the head and flex the knees high over a bolster. Fold a single steam pack, wrap it in a towel, and lay it over the patient's upper chest for 15 minutes. Remove the last one, and after using a vigorous cold friction rub on the hot area, apply a fresh hot pack. Use three changes. Finish with a mild shower, a sponge bath, or an alcohol rub. Repeat daily until recovery. Use a heating compress to the chest each night.

Good hydration is essential in treating bronchitis. Every time the patient coughs during the night a large swallow of water should be taken. Eventually the water will soothe and lubricate the surfaces and stop the irritation. Water is a good cough medicine.

For congestion of the respiratory tract, a hot foot bath with fomentations to the chest and hot drinks and plenty of blankets to produce sweating constitute an excellent treatment. If this is followed by a cold mitten friction, congestion is less likely to recur.

Bursitis

Bursae are small, flat, fluid-filled sacs near shoulders, elbows, hips, knees, and ankles. They assist in smooth and easy movements of these structures by cushioning and aiding muscles and tendons to glide past each other. Bursitis is an inflammation of this small sac. After middle age, the tendons are prone to degenerative changes and these sacs may begin to have calcium deposited in the area of the degenerating tendons, causing inflammation. Women get more bursitis than men because their shoulders slope more sharply. The sloping causes increased pressure. Heavy lifters and sedentary workers are most prone to bursitis. Try the following instructions:

1. Avoid injury to the joints that are especially vulnerable to bursitis. A strain, a direct blow, the stress of overweight, unusual shoulder or knee motions such as from painting, swimming, and lifting heavy objects at arm's length, may precipitate bursitis.
2. Allergies and infections elsewhere in the body may bring on bursitis. Live at a high level of health to avoid bursitis.
3. Do not allow excessive fatigue to develop while doing an unusual motion to which you are unaccustomed. When heavy objects must be taken in the hand for some distance, the best position is in front of one, using both hands to hold the object somewhat like a tray.
4. Do not allow chilling of the extremities, particularly the shoulders, which are especially vulnerable at night. Be careful to wear warm sleepwear.
5. Never begin heavy work until you have "warmed up" by doing some light work.
6. Use these treatments for bursitis:
   A. Heat applications may relieve pain.
   B. Ice packs to the painful area, especially in the acute phase, may relieve pain. Keep the ice on for about five to seven minutes. Remove for one minute, and repeat three times.

C. Place the patient in an upper-half body pack, as in bronchitis, making sure the upper edge is above the shoulders. Place a single steam pack over the shoulder. Cover the pack with plastic to retain heat, keeping steam out of the patient's face, and leave it in place and hot for 20 minutes. Replace with another hot one (no cold), then a third, covering a period of one hour. Finish with a shower, sponge bath, or alcohol rub. Repeat this treatment daily until the pain is gone. Early mild cases clear up in a day or two. Chronic or severe ones may require three weeks or more.

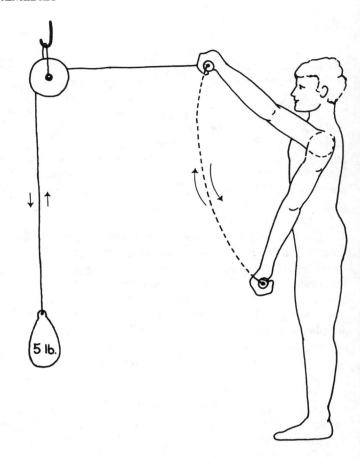

D. Hot and cold compresses are sometimes helpful in relieving the inflammation. Use three minutes of hot compresses as hot as can be tolerated, followed immediately by twenty seconds of ice water compresses. Repeat four times. Give the treatment three or four times daily.

E. Do not use deep massage as it may increase inflammation. Superficial stroking will be beneficial.

F. A short period of complete rest for the part may decrease the inflammation. A sling may be worn with much comfort. Do not prolong the period of inactivity, as a stiff joint may result.

G. Exercises: Use after any hot or cold treatment:
   1. Wall-walking exercise: Face the wall at arm's length and lean into your hands placed against the wall. Starting slightly above the level of the waist, walk hand over hand as high as you can reach without pain. As you make progress, reach higher each time before pain or tightness stops you. Repeat the exercise four times daily.
   2. A small pulley rigged up over the head with a two to five pound weight attached is helpful after the acute phase is over. Pull the arm down by the side and let the weight pull the arm over the head. Start with five to ten pulls and work up to 50 three times a day.
   3. A bicycle wheel with a small handle attached and mounted shoulder-high can be used to good advantage to get a good range of motion of the shoulder, avoiding a "frozen shoulder."

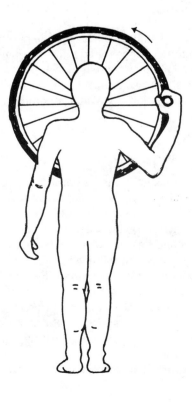

Cancer

Recent reports have appeared in many medical journals regarding the treatment of carcinomatosis (widespread cancer) with fever treatments up to 107° F. maintained for many hours, or refrigeration to 85° F., stabilizing near that level for several days. Fever treatments for cancer have been used in this century in the second and fourth decades, and increasingly from the 1960's to the present time. Both hyperthermia and hypothermia as a means of selectively destroying malignant cells have received increased attention since the 1960's. Moderate general levels of hyperthermia, 105° to 107°; and high local levels, 105.8° to 110° (41° to 43.3° C.), which can be tolerated by the host, have been demonstrated by abundant laboratory and clinical evidence to regularly effect a delay in tumor growth and often a complete regression, occasionally with permanent control of the tumor.[118] Local, regional, or systemic hyperthermia can be effective against cancer. The eradication of tumor by a single brief exposure to heat indicates that both the aerobic and the hypoxic cells have been inactivated. Suppression of DNA and protein synthesis, reduction in oxygen consumption, and labilization of lysozymes all occur with moderate hyperthermia. Effect of heating is strongly correlated with temperature level and with length of time the high temperature is maintained. An increase in temperature by one degree Celsius reduces the time for a specific response from a cell by a factor of two.

Metastatic tumors were treated with systemic hyperthermia by Stafford Warren in 1935.[119] They exhibited marked, although usually short-lived, regression of tumor and improvement of symptoms. One patient had subcutaneous masses over the flank and back. These masses completely regressed, although there was one tumor in the scapular region which diminished only to half size. There was a metastasis in the brain of this same patient which showed good response to the course of treatment, but recurred five months later. The patient died at ten months but there was at that time no evident regrowth of the disease of the flank.

In 22 patients who had malignancy of the extremities treated with perfusion hyperthermia, there was marked regression noted in nearly all instances, even if the regression did not last long in some patients. The treatment was at rectal temperature 106.7° F. (41.5° C.) for two hours and forty-five minutes.

George Crile, using a malignant tumor transplanted into the foot of young adult mice, showed that the majority could be cured by heat. For each degree Celsius rise in temperature the time required to achieve a majority-cured effect was reduced by a factor of two. If the foot was simply immersed in a water bath at 43.5° C. for 55 minutes the cure was effected in the majority of the mice, and the extremity saved. If the time was increased to 115 minutes, the majority of the mice lost the affected foot.

There are extensive reports in the medical literature, and adequate personal experience to substantiate occasional dramatic regression of cancer in patients who have incidentally had a severe febrile disease, such as typhoid. Tumor cells are more sensitive to hyperthermia than normal cells. Both hypoxic and aerobic tumor cells are inactivated by heat. There is a reduced blood flow to tumors compared to that of healthy tissues, being only 2-15% of that of adjacent body tissues. The larger the tumor the greater the reduction in blood flow to it. Tumors, consequently, absorb enough heat to self-destruct, whereas healthy tissues dissipate the heat by the circulation.

We can now say that there is abundant evidence, both laboratory as well as clinical, that the application of levels of hyperthermia that can be tolerated by normal tissue cells will result in regularly delaying growth or completely regressing the tumor, sometimes producing a permanent control of the tumor. All cultures of tumor cells in one study exhibited a death rate of 95% after two hours at 42.5° C. (107.7°). All normal cells under the same heat exposure showed a death rate of only 43%. The normal cells most severely damaged at 24 hours after exposure to heat, showed rapid repair if they survived 24 hours. In contrast, tumor cells at 24 hours did not show the ability to undergo repair; rather, they increasingly enlarged and underwent degenerative changes and death.[120]

Heat at 42° C. (107.5°) exerts an inhibitory effect on oxygen intake in rabbits. Normal host tissue cells are unaffected by the elevated temperature, but the tumors show an 80 to 95% reduction in volume with marked necrosis of tumor cells. Later macrophage invasion and replacement by fibrosis become evident. A 50% survival rate occurs in animals if only local heating is used; but only 30% of those treated with total body heating survive.[121] It should be tried in leukemia to apply the most intense heat to the flat bones, breast bones, ribs, hip bones, and spine, and less intense heat to the extremities. The older literature indicates that the destruction of tumors in man and animals requires temperatures in excess of 40° C. (104°). Recently, human neoplastic cells in tissue culture showed irreversible heat injury at only 42° C. (107.5°) and above.

Some studies indicate, however, that even if malignant cells are not killed by the heat, they are rendered incapable of reproducing themselves after having been heated to lesser temperatures. Within 24 hours of total body immersion, there is rapid necrosis and lysis of tumor cells. The most responsive tumors are malignant melanomas, fibrosarcoma, chondrosarcoma, osteogenic sarcoma, and squamous carcinoma. Rapid absorption of necrotic tumor tissue causes renal or cardiovascular complications in some patients. Stehlin noted the radiologic disappearance of lung metastases following the treatment of the primary tumor by heat. The presence of large numbers of macrophages has been consistently noted after heat therapy.[122]

Fourteen patients with a variety of metastatic malignancies were treated with total body heat, raising the rectal temperature to 41.8° C. (107.2°) for a maximum of four hours. Four patients showed tumor responses; one with colon cancer metastatic to the liver had a 40% tumor regression that lasted a year. Another with melanoma had 90% regression over ten months but treatment did not seem to halt metastases to bone. A patient with a large abdominal mass experienced 50% regression over eight months. Another had a rectal cancer that metastasized to the liver, showing 40% regression at four months.[123]

Dr. James Larkin used fever treatments for cancers of the lungs, breasts, stomach, kidney and skin. Fourteen of the 20 patients were considered hopeless, but showed 50% regression of the cancers after 2 hours at 108°. Treatment was given three times at one week intervals, under light general anesthesia. Six patients survived between 11 and 22 months. There was no central nervous system damage in his group, but the heart and liver seemed to be limiting organs. Some of the patients developed acidosis or leukocytosis. These responses may be a part of the beneficial results of the fever treatments. In 15% of patients he observed cardiac arrhythmias. Surface burns occured in 15% but he felt better padding would have prevented the burns. There was a mortality rate of 5% from massive tumor necrosis and fluid imbalance. Apparently the fever treatments cause injury to all cells, but tumor cells lack the ability of normal cells to repair themselves properly.[124]

Leveen believes that heating tumor antigens modifies the antigen in such a way as to stimulate the immunity of the individual. Certain mice who received heated cancer cells showed greater protection against implantation of tumor cells than did mice who received unheated tumor cells.[125] It may be that moderate heating of patients with cancers gives a better resistance to cancer because of the modification of the tumor antigen.

Cooling the patient was shown to have an enhancing effect on the treatment of mammary tumors in rats. Both general body cooling in a cool chamber, and locally applied cold to chill a tumor, seem to be beneficial. Greater benefit could be seen if cooling of the tumor immediately preceded or followed a heating treatment.[126]

Liver biopsy specimens from three patients during treatment of advanced malignant disease by elevation of body temperature using external heat were studied by light and electron microscopy. The liver cells showed slight swelling, nuclear alterations, and by electron microscope a large number of autophagic vacuoles, dilatation of golgi elements, endoplasmic reticulum and large cytoplasmic vacuoles. One individual developed jaundice 24 hours after hyperthermia.[127]

Chickenpox

At the beginning of the illness, a deep, quite warm bath for 15 minutes brings out the pox rapidly, makes the lesions get smaller and fade faster. Observe the usual care to keep the bowels open, the diet light and the patient reasonably quiet and sheltered. Use a spinal pack daily to stimulate the circulation and white blood cell activity, and to soothe the patient. It is not necessary to keep the patient bedfast, but just quiet. Prevent scratching the lesions and watch the pox for infection. Should it occur, combat infection in the pox in the same manner as for impetigo.

Cholera

There are two objectives in the treatment of cholera, fluid and mineral replacement and detoxification. Give a heaping tablespoon of powdered charcoal every 1-2 hours during the heaviest diarrhea, and try to stay ahead of water losses by copious drinking, intravenous administration or subcutaneous injections. To prevent potassium depletion use 6-8 ounces of green coconut water per liter of stool produced. If green coconut water is not available, tomato juice should be tried. Cholera patients can usually take fluids by mouth.[128] Frequent fomentations to the abdomen can be helpful.[129] [130]

Chorea (St. Vitus Dance, Sydenham's Chorea)

About one to six weeks following a streptococcal infection such as "strep throat" or streptococcal impetigo there is sometimes the onset of a secondary illness which may manifest itself in one of three ways: acute glomerulonephritis (Bright's disease), rheumatic fever with or without heart involvement, or a neurological disorder called chorea. The latter is recognized by inappropriate movements of the extremities or head. It is almost always seen only in childhood, before the age of 20 years. A child may jump from his chair or make writhing movements with his hands and arms while exhibiting involuntary tic-like movements of the head.

Fever therapy is the most effective way of controlling an attack of chorea. Raise the oral temperature to 101° to

103° and maintain this level for 30 minutes up to four hours each day for one week, the higher the temperature the shorter the time. The choreiform movements reduce daily. For this disorder, we do not use the very high temperature generally reported in the medical literature.

In a two year study, 45 patients with Sydenham's chorea were treated with artificial fever sessions of 105° to 105.4° rectally lasting for 2½ hours. The average number of treatments was 12.6, the average number of hours being 32.9, and the average time under treatment 22.3 days. Excellent recovery was seen in the majority of cases. There were only four recurrences during the two years. There was an incidence of prior carditis in 42.4% but this condition did not interfere with the treatments and the majority of the patients were benefited. Associated delirious episodes were infrequent during the treatments.[131]

Ninety-nine children in two groups were given fever therapy for chorea and compared with 60 patients who did not receive this treatment. For 48 of the treated patients the observation period was 1-3 years. For 51 of the treated patients the observation period was 4-6 years. The most striking finding was the higher incidence of polyarthritis and deaths from heart disease in both observation periods among the untreated cases. None of the treated cases observed from 1-3 years had aortic lesions, whereas one of the untreated patients did. Aortic disease developed in one patient in the second group observed from 4-6 years, whereas 6 in the untreated group (37 patients) had organic heart disease. In the treated group 6.6% developed acquired heart disease, whereas 46% of the untreated group developed acquired heart disease.[132]

Colds

1. The first objective in the treatment of a cold is to prevent its entrenchment by early therapy. Sometimes quick action at the first suggestion of a cold will be successful in nipping it in the bud. When symptoms are first noted, take deep breathing exercises. Inhale deeply and hold the breath for a slow count of 20. Exhale deeply and hold it for a slow count of 10. Repeat 40-50 times (this is work!). Have fresh air, but no drafts. Drafts chill body tissues unhealthfully. This exercise should be done at the first sign of a cold, even while at work or in the car, and continued through the duration of the cold several times daily. It encourages good circulation to the upper respiratory passages, and will often head off a cold.

2. Immediately, within 10 or 20 minutes of the first symptoms, put the feet in hot water, kept continually hot for 20 minutes. Then run cold water over the feet,

dry them, and cover them well or go to bed for half an hour.

3. Keep the bowels open. An enema taken at the first hint of the onset of symptoms will often prevent the development of a cold. Repeat the enema every 6-12 hours while symptoms last.

4. Get plenty of vigorous exercise, as much as can be tolerated without danger of sore muscles. If toxicity develops—headache, painful muscles and bones, weakness and fever—substitute hydrotherapy for exercise as the primary mode of treatment.

5. Drink plenty of water, enough to keep the urine quite pale. Remember that water may be lost by sweating, from increased exercise, fever, heating treatments, nasal and bronchial secretions, and by vomiting and diarrhea. Extra water must be taken to replace water lost by any of these routes.

6. Eat sparingly and only on the usual meal-time schedule. Take no juice between meals. Use no sugar, honey or very sweet fruit. Sweets reduce the immune response and may encourage the growth of viruses. Viruses replicate by the use of phosphosugars; avoiding sugar may make less phosphosugar available for their growth. Eat whole grain breads and cereals. Take foods that contain plenty of vitamins A and C. The B vitamins come from whole grains. Sunshine can produce all the vitamin D needed. Try to get some sun exposure every day. Fat also cuts down on the immune response, as well as the aggressive activity of the white blood cells. It is well to eliminate all free fat: margarine, mayonnaise, cooking oil, and fried foods.

7. Take six charcoal tablets three times daily between meals, for three days. If the throat is sore, or there are mouth ulcers, allow the charcoal to dissolve in the mouth to constantly bathe the inflamed areas.

8. Keep a regular schedule for bedtime and arising time. Take midday naps if needed. Avoid exhaustion from long hours and loss of sleep.

9. Take a hot nasal irrigation at 110° to 115° for 20 minutes (see instructions). It will often cure a cold. It is good to use an irrigation rather than nose drops as nose drops cause "rebound" nasal congestion. Use hot water to which one level teaspoon of salt has been added for each pint of water, accurately measured with a cup. Pour the hot saline into the palm and snuff it up into one nostril. It can be caught at the back of the throat and expectorated. Repeat five times before treating the other nostril. Alternate back and forth for a minimum of ten minutes.

10. Use a hot water gargle for ten minutes four times daily if needed for sore throat or earache. Take a 15 minute hot half bath, followed by a cold water pour

---

and skin friction with a dry towel for general symptoms of muscle and joint aches. Apply a sinus pack for sinus congestion or runny nose.

11. Apply a heating compress to the throat or chest as needed for sore throat or cough. This is an important treatment. Even small increases in temperature markedly decrease viral multiplication.

12. Keep the feet, hands, neck and ears warmly clothed, both day and night. Avoid the use of caffeine beverages (coffee, tea, colas). Caffeine causes constriction of the blood vessels and reduces blood flow to the hands, feet, and lining passages of the nose and throat. There is a reflex mechanism between the hands and feet and the nasal mucous membranes. The hands and feet need to be kept warm at all times. The point cannot be overemphasized that the blood flow to the nasal structures falls promptly as the temperature of the extremities falls. It is this mechanism that accounts for the low resistance to viral infection of the chilled person.

13. Do not sleep with the face covered; surveys show that 20% of Americans sleep with the face covered. Wear a nightcap and scarf for the neck if needed. Sleep in plenty of fresh air, but avoid drafts.

14. Keep the bedroom at 65° to 68° F. Avoid getting overheated, particularly sitting in a room which is too hot, as this causes dilatation of the blood vessels in the lungs with a resulting congestion and loss of resistance. Avoid sweating unless you take a shower or soon change into dry clothing, to avoid chilling from being damp.

15. A daily bath fortifies against colds, especially if it is a cool bath. Taking drugs promotes colds.

Conjunctivitis

Use small, ice cold compresses that are changed every two or three minutes for half an hour, discontinued for 30 to 60 minutes and reapplied for half an hour. Occasional applications of heat may enable the patient to continue the ice cold compresses more comfortably. During the cold applications to the eyes, a derivative effect may be produced by applying heat to the sides of the face and the chin and mouth. If the conjunctivitis becomes chronic, change the treatment to alternating hot and cold compresses—three minutes of hot compresses, and 30 seconds of cold compresses, repeated four times. Saline irrigation may be used to cleanse the eyes, if necessary, using the same procedure as for nasal irrigations. A charcoal poultice taped over the eyes at night may be helpful.

Constipation

If constipation is due to a lack of tone in the colon, give a small cool injection of water into the rectum with a bulb syringe using cool tap water. Hold for one minute, then return the water and a normal bowel movement usually follows easily. An abdominal massage is helpful in these cases as described in the massage section of this book. A cool sitz bath at 75° for 3-8 minutes taken with the feet kept out of the water and the hips submerged at least half or more in the cool water is helpful. Repeat this treatment daily before the desired time for the bowel movement.

For constipation due to a spastic colon, use a small warm or lukewarm enema from a bulb syringe (2-3 ounces are usually sufficient), warm or hot compresses to the abdomen, and a full bath at 107° for 12-20 minutes.

Coughs (see Bronchitis)

Cramps, Leg

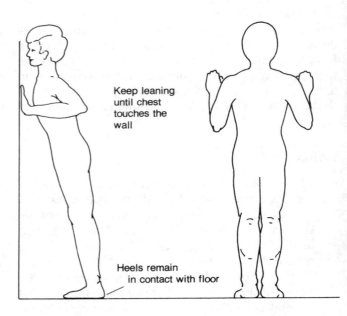

Keep leaning until chest touches the wall

Heels remain in contact with floor

Following a hot bath, stand facing a wall, toes placed 24 inches from the wall *keeping the heels always in contact* with the floor, lean into the wall until a stretch is felt in the calves. Hold for 10 seconds, release for 5 seconds and repeat 3 times. The leg stretch maneuver will usually help both leg cramps and low back pain if faithfully performed 2 or 3 times daily for four weeks.[274]

Cricks in Neck and Back

Neck pain from being cramped, from sitting in a draft, or that which follows a virus infection, may be treated with a fever treatment in a bathtub, bringing the mouth temperature up to 101° for about 10 minutes. After an hour of reacting in bed, apply an upper half body pack to the base of the skull. Shape the upper edge of the pack to the curve of the neck and up beside the ears. Leave it in place 20 to 25 minutes. Finish off either of these hot treatments with a brief cold mitten friction or cool shower. Massage the neck and shoulders to well below the bottom edge of the shoulder blades and far out on the sides with firm upward strokes until the pain and muscle spasm are gone. Spastic muscles are recognized because they are tighter than nearby muscles and have a "mass-of-tight-cords" consistency.

Next, stand at the head of the treatment table, patient face up and fully relaxed by the treatments. With your left hand on the left jaw and your right hand on the right temple, turn the head to full extension to the left, patient looking over the left shoulder. Then give the head a gentle but firm continued turn to the left, using a little pressure on the right temple to hyperextend the head about one inch beyond its natural stopping place. There should usually be no cracking sound heard. Repeat on the opposite side. This treatment loosens the pressure on the base of the skull, increases the circulation to the tendons and joints of the entire neck, and reflexively increases lymph drainage. All of these tend to relax spastic muscles.

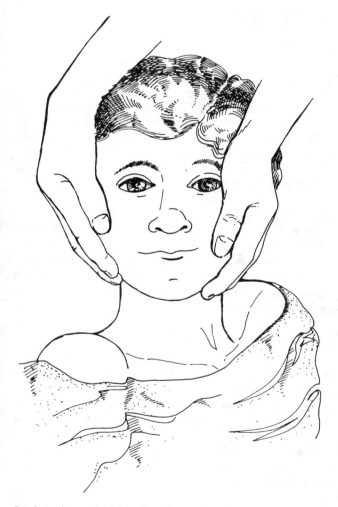

Crick in the neck. After the relaxing hot treatment, gently lift the head, apply a slight traction, and turn the head back and forth to encourage complete relaxation and confidence that you are controlling the head. With the right hand on the right temple, the left hand on the left jaw, easily rotate the head to its full extension toward the right; then hyperextend the head by firmly continuing the pressure for an inch or so.

Cystitis

Use hot fomentations alone, or alternating with brief cold compresses accompanied by much friction. Cover the low abdomen and upper thighs with the fomentation, keeping it hot continuously for eight minutes, then 20 to 30 seconds of cold. Repeat three or four times. A hot sitz bath may be substituted. A heating pad or heat lamp centered over the suprapubic area may be used continuously between other treatments.

Give buchu or other diuretic tea, 1 cup per hour during the acute phase until symptoms subside—usually about four to five hours. The diet should be carefully controlled: no sugar or other concentrated sweeteners, no oil, no caffeine or other methylxanthines (found in coffee, tea, colas and chocolate), no pepper or other spices, alcohol, baking soda or baking powder products, and only two meals daily—breakfast and a mid-day meal. No food or drink between meals except plenty of water and clear herb teas.

Dental Care

1. Use a round toothpick or dental floss after each meal to prevent periodontal disease (pyorrhea).
2. It is generally said that the teeth should be scaled and polished at least once a year, but reliable dentists point out that the use of dental floss and a soft bristle tooth brush allow longer periods between professional cleanings for most people.
3. Broken tooth—If it is not bleeding and no red spot develops on the gum to indicate an abscess, leave it alone. A sharp and jagged edge may require sanding or polishing.

4. Tooth loosened accidently with or without severing the nerves—Replace the tooth, put pressure to restore the "bite" (occlusion). If the nerve is not severed, this measure may restore the tooth. If the nerve is severed, consult a dentist for a root canal.

Dysmenorrhea

The treatment for painful menstruation should take two courses, one course to be followed before the period begins, and the second to be instituted if the menstrual period turns out to be painful.

No treatment for dysmenorrhea will be effective unless the extremities are kept quite warm, winter and summer. Few women are prepared to understand how warm the extremities need to be. They have no idea how to acclimatize themselves to having warm extremities without suffering what they believe to be overheating, but is actually a form of nerve reaction somewhat similar to claustrophobia. It is an autonomic nervous system reaction caused by overstimulation of nerve receptors on the skin. The loss of a large quantity of heat from the skin surface, or the presence of even a minor degree of chilling results in a pelvic condition involving muscular contractions and impeded circulation of lymph and blood that promotes painful menstruation. After several months the pain will subside if adequate, loose, warm clothing and a proper diet are combined with vigorous exercise and a regular and well-ordered life style.

The hot enema, a hot vaginal irrigation (douche), or a hot tub bath are all beneficial, along with a cold compress to the head and neck if sweating begins during the treatment. Follow any of these treatments with a hot foot bath. Begin the treatments four to seven days before the menstrual period is expected and discontinue about 12 hours before the expected onset. If the menstruation is again painful, the hot treatments may be restarted after the onset of the period. For acute discomfort after the period begins, hot fomentations, the revulsive sitz, and the hot vaginal irrigation (douche) are the most valuable measures.

Another type of treatment may be given as a preventive within the five days before the period is due, or even after the first signs appear that the menstrual flow has begun. Place the patient in a lower-half body pack, and lay a thick and very hot pack across the lower abdomen for twenty minutes. Remove and apply a cold friction rub. Repeat three times. Finish with a neutral or slightly warm bath. Many find much benefit from a fast the day before the period begins, with bread and fruit only on the day of the onset of the period.

Earache (Otitis Media)

Deliver heat to the ear from a table or desk lamp, or by sitting in a closed car parked in such a way that the sun can shine on the painful ear for half an hour or more, to reduce pain. Other methods to deliver heat are a hot fomentation, a partly filled hot water bottle, a heating pad, or hot salt or sand bag (oven heated). Hot gargles for ten to twenty minutes, and charcoal tablets held in the mouth may help earaches. A hot foot bath may quickly reduce the pain of earache. A charcoal poultice secured over the ear with an ace bandage should be used every night until the earache heals. Use the same treatment for mastoiditis, as it is a part of the same disease process.

Encephalitis

See Meningitis

Fevers

In vigorous young adults with fevers a hot half bath is a useful treatment. The patient should enter the tub with water at 104°, raised after half a minute to 111°, and held there for 10 to 15 minutes. Keep the face generously sponged with cold water and an ice cap to the head. Keep a thermometer in the mouth and discontinue the treatment if the mouth temperature exceeds 104.6°, or if the pulse exceeds 150. Finish the treatment with a cold shower for 10 to 20 seconds followed by a brisk rubdown with a coarse towel. Some prefer a cold mitten friction to finish. Remember that successful treatments bring large quantities of blood to the surface, a condition which can cause momentary faintness. Be prepared to support the patient until the sensation passes.

For fevers of 103° and over, the water temperature and the length of time spent in the bath should be less— the higher the fever the shorter the time. The objectives of treatment are the reversal of the heat conservation gear to the heat dissipation gear, and the stimulation of the immune system. As soon as blood comes to the skin surface, any degree of sweating is observed, or the person becomes comfortably relaxed in the bath, and begins to breathe deeply, one can assume that the objectives are accomplished and the bath may be terminated. For high temperatures in infants under six months, as brief a bath as 30 seconds followed by a 5 second cold water pour and a brisk frictioning of the skin with a dry towel, may be successful in bringing down a fever. If the treatment is long enough, a child and most adults will sleep after the treatment and will awaken with the fever reduced or entirely gone. The treatment can be repeated in infants and children as often as every two hours, but only once daily

HOT BATHS FOR FEVERS[127]

Keep the face and head cool. Follow all baths with 30-60 minutes reaction in bed.

Age of Patient	0-3 years	4-7 years	8-12 years	13-19 years	20 up
Initial Oral Temperature	99°-103°	99°-103°	99°-103°	99°-103°	99°-103°
Initial Water Temperature	106°	106°	106°	106°	106°
Water Temperature After 30 Seconds	110°	110°	110°	111°	112°
Length of Bath	3 min.	7 min.	12 min.	13-19 min.	20 min.

Age of Patient	0-3 years	4-7 years	8-12 years	13-19 years	20 up
Initial Oral Temperature	103° and over	103° and over	103° and over	103° and over	103° and over
Initial Water Temperature	104°	104°	104°	104°	104°
Water Temperature After 30 Seconds	104°	105°	106°	110°	111°
Length of Bath	3 min.	5 min.	5 min.	7-10 min.	10-12 min.

for baths lasting more than 10 minutes, since prolonged sweating can result in excessive mineral loss.

Gallbladder Pain

Use a lower-half body pack and a wide, heavy steam pack across the body from the armpits down. When it begins to cool (after 15 to 20 minutes) replace it with another hot one using cold between. Continue one hour, or until the pain stops.

In a case of chronic liver and gallbladder disturbance, use a lower half body pack, and alternate a thick upper abdominal steam pack with a vigorous ice rub every twenty minutes for three changes. Repeat the treatment as needed. Educate the patient about his diet: reducing diet if needed, no free fats, no free sugars, and only two meals per day. Gallstones that cause no symptoms should not be removed. If the patient will now assume a healthful program, the stones will remain "silent."

Gonorrhea

The aim of treatment is to destroy the causative organism by the heat. The gonococcal germ is quite fragile, being killed very easily by heat. In the early days of treating gonorrhea with fever, it was believed that a successful treatment required a temperature of 106° to 107° rectally for 5-10 hours, repeated one to five times at two to three day intervals.[128] Later it was recognized that repeated shorter sessions, 1/2 to 2 hours, were as effective as the long sessions. It is possible to cure acute or chronic urethritis (with or without associated infection of the epididymis, uterus, tubes or joints) within three to four weeks and often within two or three weeks.

Those who have had extensive experience with this treatment declare that the certainty of cure is such that it can be relied upon if the symptoms completely subside. About 92% can be expected to show complete subsidence of symptoms. The other 8% are probably caused by resistant strains of gonococcus. In one series of 100 patients, about 10% were cured after one session; about 30% in two sessions; and an additional 40% after four sessions. Some cases will require up to ten treatments. It seems desirable to give two additional treatments after the gonococcus disappears from the secretions.

The average pretreatment duration of the infection in this series was three months, the shortest three days, and the longest six years. Nevertheless, fever therapy was effective in all cases. For gonococcal infections it was found that the longer the sessions, and the shorter the interval between treatments, the more prompt the response.

The patient should be given a diet high in complex carbohydrates and sodium chloride. Give a cleansing enema the evening before the treatment. The patient may be fasting before the treatment, but there should be no restriction of fluids. The patient is encouraged to drink 300 to 400 cc. of saline solution per hour during the treatment. Make up the solution by putting 2 level teaspoons of table salt to one quart of water. The pulse seldom goes above 130 per minute. Some patients sleep during part of the treatment. Return of the temperature to normal occurs spontaneously when the skin temperature is reduced. By noon the following day, the patient is allowed to eat normally and can usually carry on regular activities. On the second day the urethral secretions are examined and re-examined every three days. If all examinations are negative the patient is dismissed. Male patients are re-examined at weekly intervals for three weeks, female patients are re-examined on the first post-menstrual day after three consecutive periods. If there is no evidence of the gonococcus by smear and culture, the patient is dismissed as cured.[136]

Headache

Headaches are not of themselves a disease, but always the reflection of disorders elsewhere in the body. Bad health habits constitute one large cause of headaches. It is sometimes hard to find the cause of headaches, but a persistent search is worthwhile. For a good beginning scrutinize all habits carefully and make any necessary changes.

The allergic headache is usually a dull ache over the forehead and cheeks. The migraine headache often makes its appearance in a tense, meticulous and obsessional person. Attacks are precipitated by numerous factors other than allergies, such as overeating, gastrointestinal upsets, emotional stress, hypothyroidism, fatigue, bright or flickering lights, and foods containing any of the following: cheese, Chianti wines, chicken liver, pickled herring, monosodium glutamate, cured meats, pressed meat and pork products. High altitudes may also be a cause of headache.

The following are some suggestions that may guide the search for the cause, prevention and treatment of headaches:

Prevention:

1. Avoid all exposure to toxins (tobacco, licit and illicit drugs; caffeine in coffee, tea, colas, and chocolate, any sweet drinks; alcohol; etc.) odors, fumes, air pollution, rotting leaves or compost, or molds from shrubs or vines growing near the house. Do not breathe, eat, drink, or touch toxic materials. Some persons are very sensitive to cosmetics and perfumes. Cat and dog dander and other pet secretions or products can cause allergic headaches in some people, as can chronic bacterial or viral infections (dental problems, chronic dermatitis, nasal lesions, and chronic genitourinary tract infections). The type of colonic bacteria associated with meat eating may cause some persons to have headaches; a change in diet may be helpful to these people. Caffeine withdrawal is notorious for causing

headache. The headache often comes on 1-3 hours after taking the food, drink, or medication containing caffeine, but may sometimes not appear until 1-3 days later.

2. There must always be circulating air in the bedroom, especially at night. In the daytime, thoroughly air the bedrooms and bed clothing, throwing the covers back upon arising. Morning headaches are often the result of stale air during the night.

3. Check during sleep time for an uncomfortable bed, or chilling of the head, neck and shoulders which may become uncovered during sleep. Because of the anatomical construction of the veins in the head, chilled blood may be thrown back over the brain from chilled shoulders. Assume a comfortable position for sleeping, usually on a side.

4. Keep the extremities warm at all times. Cold skin *anywhere* is abnormal and sends an "alarm message" to the brain. Blood that would be in the large vessels of the extremities if they were warm, is driven into the trunk and head since the arteries narrow when chilled. Many people react to chilling of the extremities by an elevation of blood pressure, which may contribute to headache. Weather changes, especially cold air, can cause headaches in susceptible persons.

5. Keep a strictly regular schedule for meals, bedtime and rising time, elimination, study periods, and other major daily events. This is an essential point.

6. Never eat even so much as a peanut between meals. Take only water and plain herb teas between meals.

7. Take no rich or heavy food. Avoid too much protein, which can give the "protein hangover" or a ketosis headache.

8. Do not eat food late in the evening. It is best to dispense with the third meal, but if supper is taken, it should be only *plain* whole grain bread or simple cooked cereal and fruit taken several hours before bedtime. Meals should be at least five hours apart.

9. Use a limited quantity and variety of food at meals. Do not mix fruits and vegetables at the same meal. Milk-sugar-egg combinations tend to cause intestinal fermentation, producing toxic substances which will give susceptible persons a headache.

10. Even apart from the food-combining problem, all dairy products tend to be associated with headaches in some people. In addition to cheese

and wine, also suspect as causes of headache are chocolate, wheat, pork, beer, eggs, citrus fruits and juices, corn, onion, garlic, nuts, tomatoes, fish and peanuts.

11. As a test, for six weeks avoid known allergenic, constipating or gas-forming foods, avoid those in the list above as well as all foods of animal origin, all refined foods, all types of beans and soy products, apples, and the "nightshades" (tomatoes, potatoes, eggplant and peppers).

12. Check the intestinal transit time by taking as a marker four charcoal tablets, or one tablespoon of sesame seed swallowed whole. Time how long the marker takes to completely clear the colon. Keep the time under 30 hours by using whole grains, extra bran, and raw fruits and vegetables.

13. Practice deep breathing. Congestion of the head can be relieved thereby. (The method is described under treatment for colds.)

14. Learn to maintain good posture while standing, sitting, walking, lying, etc.

15. Exercise from one to five hours daily out-of-doors.

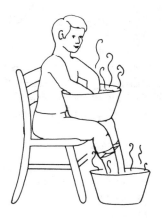

Treatment

1. At the very beginning of a headache, take a hot mustard immersion bath to both the feet, hands, and arms to the elbows with a cold compress to the head for 20 minutes or more. Use one teaspoon of dry mustard to one to two gallons of hot water.

2. If the headache develops after the initial treatment use the next step. Alternate hot and cold to the head using the following procedure: hot water bottle or hot fomentation to the base of the head and cervical spine, ice water compress to the face and temples, ears and forehead. After three minutes exchange the hot with cold compresses, and the cold with hot compresses. Give three complete sets of hot and cold. Always use with a moderately hot foot bath, 103° to 106°.

3. Some headaches may continue unabated, or recur. If so, try the following treatment: Simultaneous hot and cold to the head; ice bag to the base of the skull, a second ice bag to the forehead, and ice bags or ice compresses over both carotids in the neck; a simultaneous application of hot compresses on the face, covering the ears and forehead. Maintain the treatment from five to forty-five minutes, determined by the reaction of the patient. If the headache abates quickly, discontinue the treatment, but continue even for several hours if it persists. Always use with a moderately hot foot bath, 103° to 106°.

4. If nervousness is a feature of the headache, take a neutral bath for 30 to 45 minutes. The water temperature should be tepid or lukewarm. Blot skin dry—no brisk rubbing. Dress quietly.

5. Drink a cup of red clover tea or catnip tea at the onset of a headache.

6. Induce vomiting with the finger if undigested food is fermenting in the stomach. The patient usually recognizes a spoiled, acid, or fermented taste in the mouth or about burped materials or gasses.

7. Give enemas until clear, using hot water or charcoal water.

8. Take a brisk walk, *extremities well protected* from dampness or chilling, head up, shoulders back, breathing deeply to relieve congestion.

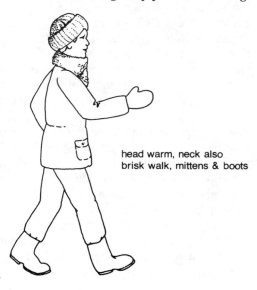

head warm, neck also
brisk walk, mittens & boots

9. At the first sign of a migraine—dizziness, blurred vision, black or colored spots in the visual field, nausea, etc., try the following procedure:
   A. Seat the person in a chair with the head hanging between the knees.
   B. Apply a gentle flow of very cold water to the base of the skull, allowing it to flow forward through the hair over the scalp for *30 seconds*. Catch the run-off water in a pan placed between the feet. Briefly dry the hair and scalp by blotting with a towel.
   C. Allow the person to sit up promptly after the water pouring procedure, elevating the feet on a stool. Direct a stream of cold water, under pressure if possible, to the soles of the feet for 1½ to 2 minutes. If water under pressure is not available, use one quart of ice water poured over the feet for 60 seconds.
   D. After the cold water pour, apply pressure to the temples with the heels of the hands, exerting as much pressure as can be generated between the palms, for two to five minutes. *Gradually* reduce the pressure—do not suddenly let go—using about one minute to accomplish the full release.
   E. Repeat every two hours until the headache is gone.

10. The tension type headache is best treated with a steam pack on the shoulders and back of the neck for twenty minutes, followed by massage of the neck and shoulders and finger stroking over the forehead and back through the hair to relax the scalp. A simultaneous hot foot bath will assist with the derivative effect.

11. Sometimes there is some distortion in the position of the vertebrae, and it is helpful to use gentle manual traction to the neck: just maintain a sustained pull for one to ten minutes on the head. Hook the fingertips around the base of the skull and the angles and undersurfaces of the jaw.

12. During any prolonged treatment routine for headache, especially if all measures have been applied but the headache continues, sit for a while at the head of the patient and simply lay one hand on the forehead and place the other hand at the base of the skull at the neck. Even this simple touch can often be comforting.

13. In treating migraine it is sometimes necessary to go through your entire armamentarium of treatments, apply Number 12 above, and start over.

Sometimes a second application is more effective than the first time, sometimes less.

Heart Tonic

For assisting a failing or weak heart a number of simple stimuli may be helpful: (1) Very hot and short applications of 3-7 minutes, over the heart while applying alternating hot and cold applications to the spine; (2) hot water drinking; (3) the small cold enema (see instructions elsewhere); and (4) a very short application of cold to almost any part of the body, but especially to the face and chest.

Hemorrhage

To stop bleeding with hot or cold applications, the temperature of the water must be either very hot (115° to 125°), or very cold (32° to 40°). An even hotter temperature may be used and is more efficient in stopping hemorrhage, but must be carefully regulated. At 127° to 130° no greater than 30 second exposure is allowed (see chart). Direct applications of heat to stop bleeding are generally more useful than cold in nosebleeds, menorrhagia (excessive menstrual bleeding); postpartum hemorrhage, a blood ooze from denuded surfaces, and bladder hemorrhage. Hot water packs at 115° to 120° placed on the spinal column from the lower thoracic to the sacral region have arrested postpartum hemorrhage.[137] "Hot lap packs" have been used successfully in surgery for generations in the treatment of bleeding from large surface areas, C-sections, and mechanical injuries.

Precautions:

Most people cannot remove themselves from a shower, tub, or pan of hot water in less than one-half second. After a slip in the shower, or in the case of the neurologically handicapped, 10 to 20 seconds might be required to react to hot water and remove oneself. Tap water temperatures should be kept below 130° (55° C.), and 135° (57° C.) is definitely dangerous if small children or elderly people are in the home.

Burns at Specific Temperatures

Temperature	Length of Direct Exposure	Degree of Skin Burn Possible
158° (70° C.)	1 second	Full thickness of skin
149° (65° C.)	2 seconds	Full thickness of skin
140° (60° C.)	3-5 seconds	Full thickness of skin
135° (57° C.)	10 seconds	Full thickness of skin
133° (56° C.)	15 seconds	Full thickness of skin
127° (53° C.)	60 seconds	Full thickness of skin
124° (51° C.)	3 minutes	Full thickness of skin

A. Nosebleeds

Cold applications may be put on the upper spine at the base of the skull for checking nosebleeds. Also try placing the hands in ice water, or the feet in cold water.

B. Lung Hemorrhage

For pulmonary hemorrhage place a very cold compress over the front of the chest and very hot fomentations between the shoulder blades, taking care to cover both the lower cervical and upper thoracic region. Do not extend the hot packs below the lower edge of the shoulder blades. Continue the hot fomentations and cold compress for six minutes. Keep the patient in the upright or slightly reclining position; move the patient as little as possible, and combat sweating and a sensation of overheating by sponging the face or using a gentle breeze from a fan. Do not permit the slightest degree of chilling as that sends blood to the internal organs, including the lungs. A more reclining position can be assumed as the hemorrhage subsides.

C. Stomach Hemorrhage

For gastric hemorrhage, small lumps of ice may be swallowed and large ice compresses placed over the epigastrium. As long as bleeding continues the patient must be kept fasting, administering water by retention enema. The pulse and blood pressure should be carefully watched and blood replacement made if the patient vomits significant quantities of red blood. Passing black, tarry stools and vomiting "coffee-ground material" are less ominous than vomiting red blood. Do not forget that the compensatory mechanisms of the body can adjust for hemorrhage for several hours before shock appears suddenly. Vomiting as much as a cup or two of blood unmixed with food represents a medical emergency.

D. Intracranial Bleeding

In stroke, the ice cap and the ice cold compresses to the head and neck are most appropriate. The standard treatment includes also the hot foot bath. The flushing of the face and the congested neck veins often seen in stroke will improve before your eyes after beginning a hot foot bath. Restlessness and agitation can be combated by cool facial sponging, cool water or ice cravat, warm steam packs to the spine or chest, and hot fomentations to the low abdomen and upper thighs. Massage, moist abdominal binder, and hot immersion arm baths are all helpful. The patient must be kept very quiet, and in a room with subdued light. Visitors are strictly forbidden.

E. Postpartum Hemorrhage

In postpartum hemorrhage a very hot compress (prepared from water at about 120°), or a hot douche at 120°, or both, may be used. The compresses may be applied to the thighs and spine and a simultaneous ice bag placed over the lower abdomen, while the hot vaginal douche is being prepared. The hot compresses must be refreshed every 30 seconds. The ice bag and hot compresses are left in place only about five or six minutes, and should be removed after this length of time as they will eventually promote reflexive arterial dilatation. Then the hot vaginal irrigation at 115° to 125° should be started if not already in progress before the compresses and ice bag are removed. The interior of the cervix and uterus may also be irrigated with the hot water. At water temperatures of 121° to 123° maintain the irrigation for only 3 minutes. At lower temperatures the irrigation can be continued for a longer period, but not prolonged past 6 minutes. Its greatest effectiveness is in the first one to two minutes. Water temperatures below 110° will not be effective to stop hemorrhage.

F. Excessive Menstrual Bleeding

Since some women respond to one treatment and some to another, it is well to have a number of treatments available for use in gynecologic conditions. For menorrhagia, use a hot vaginal douche at about 115° to 122° for one to three minutes. A hot foot bath for two minutes at 120° is often helpful along with a cold application to the low abdomen and inner thighs. A very powerful vaginal treatment is a cold tap water irrigation for six minutes. Another good treatment is that of putting the patient in a shallow sitz bath at 50° to 70° for five to fifteen minutes, the feet being placed in very hot water at the same time.

A valuable method to treat excessive menstrual bleeding is a fever treatment using an appropriate bath to elevate the temperature to 104° briefly, reduce to 101°, and hold at that level for 30 minutes. The diet should be changed to include daily a serving of the following high steroid foods: corn, apples, carrots, peanuts, sweet potatoes, tomatoes, and white potatoes. Take one tablespoon each of shredded coconut (unsweetened), and wheat germ. The herbs that are helpful are alfalfa, red raspberry, and garlic.

Hernia, Incarcerated

An incarcerated hernia is one that is "stuck," that will not reduce. It may constitute a medical emergency if not soon released, since pressure and swelling of the involved loop of bowel will eventually interfere with the blood supply to the bowel, causing irreversible damage.

An incarcerated hernia may be treated by decreasing the tone of the voluntary muscles of the abdomen through the application of heat. The patient may be allowed to rest in a mildly hot tub bath to reduce the tone of the abdominal musculature so that the hernia may be released. A deep breathing exercise should be practiced during the bath to encourage decongestion of the hernia. If cold is applied to the abdominal wall the muscles tighten as do the involuntary muscles of the gastrointestinal tract, urinary bladder, and gallbladder. By the alternating of applications of heat and cold, the blood movement through any internal organ may be influenced. Cold contracts the visceral vessels by reflex action, while heat produces the opposite effect. By the alternation of these effects a veritable pumping action may be instituted. After 3 or 4 minutes the abdominal wall is nicely relaxed. Put slight sustained pressure on the hernia with the fingers while the patient forcibly sucks in his breath and reduces the pressure in the abdomen and chest. To apply the pressure with a cold compress held firmly against the hernia may be useful. May need to repeat the procedure several times.

Hepatitis (Jaundice)

A. Acute Jaundice

Make sure of good elimination daily and copious water drinking. For the first week give a diet principally of fruit and whole grains—no nuts or coarse vegetables. Avoid entirely all free oils, free sugars, rich foods, spices, baking soda, and baking power products, caffeine, alcohol, drugs of all kinds, and more than three dishes at a meal. Confine the diet to fruits, vegetables and whole grains. Return gradually to a regular diet as recovery progresses.

Give the following treatment daily: place the patient in a lower half body pack. Apply a wide, thick steam pack over the lower chest and upper abdomen for 15 minutes, then give a thorough cold rub, another steam pack, and so on for four repetitions. Finish with a shower or a sponge bath. One treatment often suffices for the mild, acute, toxic forms of hepatitis such as in post-alcohol intoxication. The acute infectious hepatitis will take several days.

Cold water applied over the lower portion of the right chest and epigastrium are very effective in increasing liver circulation. Keep the patient on bed rest with bathroom and meal privileges until the skin loses its yellow color. Then limit the physical activity until the

bilirubin returns to normal by laboratory tests (3-5 weeks). Fewer cases of relapse and "chronic active hepatitis" apparently result if activity is limited. A little walking about the house and yard until the bilirubin is again within normal limits appears to be best, followed by a graduated exercise program as soon as the liver is functioning well. Daily sun baths are helpful in reducing jaundice.

B. Chronic Jaundice

The sweating bath is of great value, both to relieve itching and to eliminate bile. Charcoal and wheat bran are both effective in reducing the amount of bile salts that are reabsorbed into the blood from the gastrointestinal tract.

In chronic active hepatitis, artificial fever therapy two or three days a week, with fomentations over the liver on the off-days may be beneficial.

Herpes Simplex (Fever Blisters)

At the very first sign of fever blister, when there is a stinging sensation on the lip, or some indication of numbness, an ice cube should be held to the area for 60 to 90 minutes. The treatment is sufficient to completely abort the development of fever blisters in 24 hours.

Should the fever blister be completely developed before it is recognized, it is still wise to place the ice cube on the lip for 30 to 45 minutes, although the beneficial effects of completely eradicating the fever blister within 24 hours cannot be expected once the lesion is entirely developed. If there is swelling or exudate, the fever blister should be treated with hot and cold applications, using alternating fomentations and cold compresses, as described elsewhere. Give the treatment every two hours until the swelling begins to reduce. A cool compress wet with golden seal tea, or direct applications of moistened golden seal powder may be helpful in relieving pain and swelling.

Impetigo

First use a heat treatment, usually a bath is preferred, in which crusts are removed, followed by a charcoal compress in the interval between baths. Every two hours a new hot bath can be administered. Towels should be kept strictly separate so that the patient does not share a towel with any other person, and the towel used on the affected area is not used elsewhere, as the lesions tend to spread easily.

Infectious Mononucleosis

Use the same treatment as for shingles.

Influenza

The major precaution in influenza, apart from the use of ordinary therapeutic means, is protecting the patient from chilling. Close-fitting sleeping garments and bed socks with a night cap and "pneumonia jacket" may all be used to good advantage. Fresh air should be freely circulating in the sick room, but no drafts should be allowed. During treatments the room should be significantly warmer than usual, around 72°. The first treatment should be a vigorous sweat, in a warm room, with a hot foot bath. Tub baths are not best in influenza if there is the likelihood of getting chilled when transferring from the tub to the bed. After the first sweating treatment, subsequent treatments should avoid much sweating. Influenzal pneumonia is the most common serious complication, and can usually be avoided by the use of hydrotherapy and strict adherence to avoiding exposure and chilling. Cough may be relieved by drinking copious quantities of water, a heating compress, or by fomentations to the upper chest.

Insomnia (Sleeplessness)

Apply a thick, very warm (not hot) fomentation to the spine for 20 to 30 minutes, (the patient may lie on it if desired). Remove the fomentation, dry the skin, and gently return to bed. Sleep comes as a natural result of normal fatigue, and in most cases all that is necessary in the treatment of insomnia is to produce this normal fatigue by proper exercise.

A neutral bath at a temperature of 94° to 97° will aid in reducing congestion of the brain and spinal cord, a very frequent accompaniment of insomnia. A massage is often effective as are catnip and hops tea. Remember that very hot or very cold treatments are stimulatory for many, and arouse rather than sedate. The same can be said of brisk exercise. But for some persons a cold mitten friction, starting with an already warm patient, is effective for inducing sleep. A long (20-30 minute) hot bath at 104° will help some. All treatments for insomnia should include 10 to 20 slow, deep breaths of fresh air while the patient is comfortably relaxed in a nice warm bed.

Iritis

Iritis is a painful and often serious inflammation of the iris; it may be due to a virus infection or it may be associated with such systemic diseases as rheumatoid arthritis or tuberculosis. It has a tendency to recur frequently and to become chronic. It is characterized by pain which is often deep and severe, in contradistinction to the mild or moderate irritation and burning of conjunctivitis. There is often intense redness and engorgement of conjunctival vessels and photophobia (aversion to light). We have treated severe cases with artificial fever therapy using either the Russian bath or heated whirlpool. In every case there has been subsidence of the acute attack, without complications. The number of treatments has varied from one to six. It has not been necessary to use drug dilatation of the pupil as is commonly prescribed with these treatments.

Kidney Stones

Very large, very hot fomentations are needed and should be applied quickly, while the heat is still almost unbearable. Maintain the hot application, keeping it hot with hot water bottles or heating pad. Keep the head cool by cold compresses. See section on kidney stone pack.

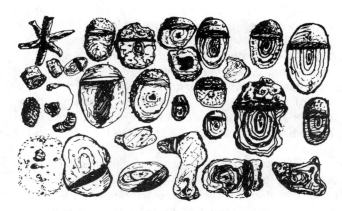

Various Human Stones

Malaria

Malaria is caused by Plasmodium, a parasite introduced into the blood stream by a bite from an infected female Anopheles mosquito, the one that stands on her head to bite. The parasite enters a red blood cell and multiplies until it forms a whole rosette of new parasites, and bursts the cell. At the time a crop of red cells begin to burst, the patient starts having chills. When the red cells rupture, all the new malaria parasites are set free in the bloodstream, and each one immediately searches for a new red cell to inhabit. The patient continues to have a fever while the parasites are free in the plasma. Even a small number of parasites are capable of provoking a high fever with shaking chills. Any successful attack on malaria has to be made during this parasite migration phase.

An excellent treatment begins with a hot water enema followed by two quick fomentations of three minutes each to the abdomen. As the second of these two fomentations is being applied, begin a cold mitten friction to the rest of the body, starting with the upper extremities, proceeding to the lower extremities, finishing the second fomentation with a cold mitten friction to the abdomen and chest, turning the patient and ending with a cold mitten friction to the back. Follow this first phase of treatment with a rest of 1 to 1¹/₂ hours.

The next portion of the treatment is alternating hot and cold fomentations, two quick ones to the spine, very hot, and about three minutes each, with one minute cold compresses following each three minute hot fomentation. When the fomentations to the spine have been completed, give a hot foot bath with alternating hot and cold spray to the liver and spleen area. The patient may stand in the hot foot bath in the shower while the hot and cold spray are being administered to the midsection. Give the hot spray at about 110° and the cold spray at about 40° to 50°.

Continue the treatment for 10 to 20 minutes. The patient should be quite warm during this part of the treatment. The second phase of the treatment ends with a vigorous cold mitten friction for five minutes while sitting in a bathtub, the water at about 70° to 80°. One may substitute a cold mitten friction in bed for a debilitated patient, or a salt glow followed by a cool cleansing shower at about 90° to 94°. At the end of the second phase the patient should rest in bed to react for 1 to 1¹/₂ hours.

Another method of treatment for malaria consists of taking the temperature every 15 minutes; at the first sign of an elevation of body temperature, put the patient into a full body pack, a Russian steam bath, a whirlpool, or a hot bathtub, to elevate the temperature to about 102° to 103°, bringing out the army of white blood cells into the blood stream to attack the parasites before they can enter new red blood cells. You probably will not catch them all the first treatment, but persevere. Be ready with a full-body pack every time the symptoms appear, whether it is every 3 days, 4 days, or at irregular intervals. Used with persistence and proper timing, this treatment will completely eradicate the disease.

The malaria drugs depress the white cells both in the bone marrow and in the blood. You are dependent on the phagocytic activity of the white blood cells to eradicate the parasites.

Mastoiditis—See Earache.

Measles (Rubeola)

Observe the usual precautions of good elimination, light diet, abundant fluids, a darkened room, and keeping the patient quiet. Protect the eyes from bright light. Instead of using aspirin or Tylenol for fever, simply sponge the child lightly with hot water or give a brief hot bath about one minute for each year of the child's age, to draw the blood to the skin for cooling. Repeat every two hours as needed until the fever has finished. The treatment not only cools the blood but also boosts the immune system. Shelter the patient carefully, particularly avoiding chilling until recovery is complete.

Meningitis, Encephalitis

Observe the patient carefully and be careful with all treatments. Begin with a hot leg pack with ice cravat and ice cap to the head and ice bag to the base of the brain and upper spine. After this treatment is in progress, you may add fluxion to the spine using alternating hot and cold packs in a narrow strip down the spine about three to six inches wide.

The main objectives of treatment in meningitis are (1) to reduce the cerebral congestion and relieve the cerebral symptoms, and (2) to relax the muscular rigidity. Using both the derivative to the lower extremities and simultaneous cold to the head will help with the cerebral symptoms. The rigidity can be helped by warm packs or a warm bath at about 99°.

It has been shown that raising the temperature of the patient to 103° to 106° for at least 30 minutes daily for five consecutive days in an ordinary bathtub with the temperature of the bath being gradually raised to 110° causes an increase in the permeability of the blood vessels in the spinal cord. It seems likely that a greater fluxion and removal of toxins from the brain will occur with fever treatments.[139]

Neutral baths at 90° (32° C.) were given in two cases of cerebrospinal meningitis with such marked success that Dr. Worochilski recommended this treatment be widely adopted as a therapeutic measure. The effect of the first bath was surprising; the irregular pulse became regular, the temperature fell, the patient felt so much improved that he begged for more hot baths.[141] Dr. Osler treated meningitis with warm baths every third hour.[142] Grosse treated meningitis with hot baths beginning at 100° to 103° for one minute, then rapidly increasing to 107° for 3-6 minutes, the longer period for older children. Use no cold pour at the end unless there is difficulty breathing, in which case use water at 93°, never colder.[143] The hot foot bath with cold compress to the head and neck make a good derivative in strokes and inflammation of the brain or meninges.

Menopause

Unpleasant symptoms at the menopause may be relieved by a cool bath every morning. A woman who has made regular and persistent use of the cold bath for some years preceding the menopause is very unlikely to experience hot flashes. Precede the bath with a brush massage. Use the diet recommended elsewhere in this book for excessive menstrual bleeding. Begin a graduated exercise program that has as its objective 3-5 hours daily of vigorous outdoor work.

Mental Illness

Forms of hydrotherapy useful in treating mentally ill persons include the sedative pack (full body pack), a neutral bath or whirlpool, the warm fomentation, or wet sheet pack allowed to warm up to neutral. The latter have given far more satisfactory results than other types of hydrotherapy.

To obtain a stimulating effect, use graduated cold packs beginning mild and getting colder, followed by cold mitten friction to insure a good reaction. In one mental hospital in Illinois before the era of tranquilizers, during a 9 year period in which hydrotherapy for mental illness was being constantly developed and extended, an increasing improvement rate with more hospital discharges was experienced. During the first three year period the percentage of patients paroled and discharged was 38.2. During the second three year period there were 44.63%, and during the third 67.83%. Patients treated with hydrotherapy were found to be more comfortable, less in conflict with others, and less in restraints.[262]

The treatment of psychotic patients with either general or local applications of heat while neglecting the use of cold to the head may increase the psychotic symptoms. Dr. Henry Kefauver reports a case of manic-depressive psychosis who was being treated with a continuous neutral bath for 6 hours at 90° to 96°, beginning at 8:00 A.M. At this time his pulse was 104, and he was restless and talkative. A cold compress was applied to the forehead before the bath. In one hour the pulse rate dropped to 84. At 10:30 the patient became very excited, noisy and unmanageable, breaking through the canvas cover of the tub, and refusing further treatment. At that time the patient was immediately placed in cold wet sheet packs. On investigation it was learned that the cold compress to the head had been removed when the pulse dropped to 80. The water temperature had been increased, making it then a hot bath, raising the body temperature, and the pulse made a corresponding rise to 124. After the cold wet sheet was applied, the patient received cold to the head again, and the pulse again dropped to 80.

At that time the patient slept nearly an hour in the pack and was removed quiet and cooperative, with pulse rate around 76.[144]

A patient with schizophrenia was given a continuous neutral bath of three hours' length beginning at 96° at 8:00 A.M. The patient was excited, combative, and very noisy at the time of being placed in the tub. A cold compress was applied to the forehead and an ice cap to the back of the neck after entering the tub. He became quieter in the bath, pulse 88. A noticeable increase in restlessness and talkativeness occurred during the second hour when it was discovered that the ice cap had become warm, ice entirely melted. The patient's face had not been sponged, and the face was flushed with some perspiration showing on the upper lip. The pulse was 96 at 10:00 A.M. and water temperature 96°. Upon renewal of cold to the head, face and neck, the patient immediately began to feel more comfortable and quiet, his face lost its redness, and perspiration stopped. The patient was removed at 11:00 A.M. much quieter, with a pulse of 80.[144]

For another schizophrenic patient, catatonic type, the prescriptions included cold mitten friction, salt glows, saline baths, shampoos, needle sprays, and fan douches. The patient did not talk, was noncooperative, resistive, and antagonistic. The mittens used were made of Turkish towel material and wrung from cold water at 60°. This treatment was continued at regular intervals for about two months when the patient began to show signs of noticing things and with urging could be gotten out of bed for a short period. At that time the prescription was changed to tonic baths, salt glows three times a week, saline baths twice weekly at 97° for 30 minutes. He was given body shampoos one day a week. Hot foot baths at 104° to 110° were administered preparatory to the tonic procedures. Cold compresses were applied to the forehead prior to putting the feet in hot water. With the salt glow the cold compresses to the head were changed after treating each body section. During the saline baths the cold compresses were changed every ten minutes. After 7 months of treatment the patient was given an outside parole.

A. Tranquilizer, Natural

Fill a bathtub with water at 92° to 98°. The patient lies back in the tub, two towels are used to drape over the knees, and the shoulders and chest, so that only the head is above water. Use a bath thermometer to keep the temperature constant. Avoid drafts, distractions, and disturbing thoughts. The tranquilizing effect lasts 20 minutes or more. If the patient falls asleep he has achieved the maximal effect. If the patient is to go to bed after the treatment, he needs only to blot the skin dry. If he is to go to work, he should take a brief cool shower, or cold mitten friction, to dispel any sense of "retardation," (sluggish circulation, headache and malaise).

B. Nervousness

It should be constantly borne in mind during treatment with hydrotherapy or other means of rational therapy, that the applications must be persistently applied, and not discontinued after a brief trial. Time and patience will eventually result not only in the disappearance of symptoms, but in most instances, also in the reduction of the basic disease process. Under no circumstances is the patient to be neglected. The treatments are to be as faithfully and precisely applied as would medications or manipulations had a physician prescribed them. However, in particular diseases with aspects that may be referred to as "nerve storms," such as neuralgia, migraine, tic douloureux, nervous attacks, etc., there may be a worsening of the patient's condition during the first few days or weeks of treatment. An effort must be made to maintain the patient's courage, so that he may be induced to persevere in the program. Tell the patient, "You must expect to feel worse before you feel better." This exaggeration of symptoms, and the occasional appearance of new symptoms can be attributed to the intensity of the visceral activity set up by the strong stimulation of the nervous system produced by the hydrotherapeutic measures. Therefore, the treatments should not be considered to be disagreeing with the patient, or to indicate that he is getting worse, but rather to indicate that the effects are being observed on schedule.

There are, however, certain symptoms which may result from too great extremes in temperature, too long a duration of treatment, an excessive or incomplete reaction, or certain physiological factors. These unwanted or unpleasant effects of rational therapy may include headache, dizziness, sweating, insomnia, palpitations, nervousness, skin drying, fever blisters, taking cold, or a psychological aversion to the treatment routine.

For nervousness, place the patient on a bed of steam packs extending from the neck to the thighs, tucked up well on the sides of the neck and ribs. Maintain the packs for 30 minutes. Remove, give a shower or sponge bath, and follow with a massage. See other treatments for mental disorders.

Multiple Sclerosis

The use of cold applications in the management of spasticity or paralysis can assist patients to carry out exercise and self-care programs in a more active and func-

tional manner. Techniques for applications of the cold vary somewhat. Moist cold is more effective than a dry ice bag. Heat is not as successful in the treatment of spasticity, nor in reducing the weakness. Cold applications consisting of crushed ice wrapped in wet towels, placed over the spastic groups of muscles for ten minutes, should be followed by exercise to the muscles, or groups of muscles. The favorable effects may last for as long as 12 hours.

Another method of applying the cold is by immersion of an extremity in cold water at 50° for ten minutes followed by exercise of the part. Injuries and multiple sclerosis have been successfully treated in this way. To immerse a patient in a Hubbard tank at 80° for ten minutes can increase movement and reduce the stretch reflex. Thirty percent of patients so managed derive little or no prolonged benefits from cold therapy, but the remainder receive measurable help.

Use fever treatments in an effort to slow down the progress of the disease. Use cold baths for the temporary muscle strengthening obtained in order to prevent muscular atrophy. Since raising the temperature reduces nerve transmission briefly, various body functions such as vision, muscular strength, etc. will often be lost or diminished at specific levels during the rise in body temperature. An interesting phenomenon is that the functions are regained when the temperature is on the way down at a *higher* temperature than they were lost on the way up. Apparently there is a tolerance or benefit gained by the treatment for temperature elevations. Use a temperature level to 103° to 104° rectally, 30 to 60 minutes, three to five times weekly for about 20 treatments.

Mumps

Observe the precautions of good elimination, and light diet, and keep the patient quiet and sheltered, although not necessarily in bed, until the swelling and tenderness of the parotid gland disappear. Much vigorous activity or exposure to cold during the illness can easily cause a worsening. A daily spinal steam pack is a great help in keeping the patient quiet and the condition improving.

Parkinson's Disease

The treatment of any chronic disease must extend over long periods of time and is often unsatisfactory when the cause of the disease is unknown, as in Parkinson's disease. The need of treating their symptoms is apparent. In this condition there may be many unpleasant sensations, especially burning of the skin, as well as tremors and rigidity of muscles. The use of the continuous bath (a hammock bath in a tub of continuously running water) can relieve symptoms remarkably. Begin the bath at 92° in a well-ventilated and cool room. Some patients may want a warmer room than others, and may want the bath water at 95° or even 98°. The comfort of the patient should be consulted. Maintain the bath for about two hours and follow it with a light general massage or alcohol rub. Give the baths 5 to 6 times a week.

During the first half hour a slight fall in blood pressure and increase in pulse and respiration can be expected. Very quickly the burning and other unpleasant sensations cease. The tremors diminish or stop while in the water. Some patients are enabled to stop all medications and make permanent improvement. Others are helped only while they are actually in the bath. For these, it is quite permissible to continue the baths beyond 2 hours, even 12-15 hours as availability of personnel permits.

It is very important to combat constipation, as this condition makes both rigidity and tremors worse. The beneficial effect of the bath is the soothing of a barrage of nerve impulses from the skin which reflexively produces a calming influence to reduce the tremors and rigidity. Constipation acts similarly to send a barrage of peripheral impulses but when these impulses signal a disorder, they act as irritants and cause tremors and rigidity. Anything that will quiet nerve impulses from any part of the body will have a beneficial effect on Parkinson's disease—keeping the extremities warm both summer and winter, relieving skin problems, avoiding minor illnesses, and keeping the bowels cleansed and freely functioning.[145]

Pelvic Problems—Female Diseases

Pelvic Inflammatory Disease, Acute or Chronic Salpingitis

Pelvic inflammatory disease requires vigorous derivatives. Pain relief is usually prompt.

Hydrotherapy is effective in all pelvic conditions, including gonorrhea. The patient with ordinary bacterial salpingitis should first be given a hot vaginal irrigation at 110° to 115° of three gallons of vinegar water (1/4 cup per gallon). Next, give a hot foot bath for 10 minutes, followed by a hot hip and leg pack, then full blanket pack to produce fever while applying cold compresses, or an ice bag to the groin and suprapubic region. Finish with a cold mitten friction. Repeat twice daily until the acute inflammation subsides. Any or all of these measures used on a rotating schedule will usually be effective to relieve

pain and reduce toxicity. For chronic salpingitis use the revulsive sitz bath every day for 30 to 60 days.

Uterine Retroversion and Endometriosis

There is no cure for either of these conditions, but the treatment for the discomfort experienced in both cases is identical.

Retroversion or backward tipping of the uterus probably causes few if any symptoms. Most women who have retroversion never know about it. Most pelvic discomfort is probably due to some other cause. However, an occasional woman feels better when a pessary is being worn to brace the uterus in a forward position, or when simple hydrotherapy reduces the pelvic congestion if this condition is present.

Endometriosis consists of abnormally placed islands of endometrial glands and stroma, the tissue which normally lines the uterus. Islands of this tissue may be found in unusual places, misplaced between the rectum and vagina, around the fallopian tubes, in the uterine muscle itself, or in the ovaries. Some authorities believe the displacement of the endometrial tissue into the surrounding structures occurs when there are forceful uterine contractions during the menstrual period. The Levitical laws of the Bible prohibit sexual relations during or immediately following the menstrual period. It may be that prevention of endometrial implants was the objective of this law.

For endometriosis and retroversion, use the hot sitz bath alternating with the cold sitz bath, or hot and cold applications to the sacrum, feet and legs, accompanied by much friction. A cold mitten friction should form a part of the regimen for these cases.

In tilting of the uterus, have the patient empty the lower bowel well at bedtime. The small cold enema is useful here. She should assume a knee-chest position for five minutes, flattening out in bed afterward without rising up again. Repeat each night for several nights before the menstrual period.

Peptic Ulcer

1. Use a 24 hour fast to cut down hydrochloric acid production. Willow bark tea is helpful to stop bleeding; use in small amounts, only if the ulcer is actively bleeding.
2. Begin simple diet limited to small meals of fruit, vegetables and whole grains the second 24 hours. No fluids with meals. Chew well, take small bites, and eat slowly. Blend foods if teeth are poor. Use only three meals daily and do not eat between meals. Drink plenty of water between meals to soothe the stomach and dilute the hydrochloric acid. Remember

that hydrochloric acid is produced in response to food in the stomach, especially high protein food. We use 2 tablespoons of aloe vera juice or catnip tea as needed for pain.

3. Eliminate all irritating substances: tobacco, alcohol, caffeine, sweets, vinegar, drugs, spices, baking soda and powder, other substances which inflame the stomach and nerves, and wrong eating habits such as eating off schedule, nibbling, and poor chewing.

4. Observe strict regularity in mealtime and bedtime. Get exercise, but do not be overly enthusiastic for a few days. Take time off from work. It has been known for years that a break in one's regular routine is often beneficial for ulcer patients. You may putter around the house, stopping for a ten minute rest in bed every hour.

5. Use fomentations with alternating hot and cold to the abdomen. When a peptic ulcer is bleeding, make the fomentations very hot. These are the hottest fomentations we use, truly as hot as can be tolerated, and lasting for two minutes, followed by an ice rub or very wet ice cold compress.

6. Between fomentations, apply a poultice of equal quantities of charcoal and olive oil to the abdomen.

Phlebitis

Heat and elevation are the mainstay for phlebitis. Place a standard steam pack lengthwise under the affected limb and lay another over the limb. It should stay effectively hot for about 30 minutes, and it may be renewed if desired. Wrapping with a plastic sheet helps to prevent heat loss; a garbage bag can be used quite effectively. Follow it with a hot and cold water bath like the leg bath for varicose veins.

Where there are signs of inflammation (heat, swelling, pain and induration or hardness) along the course of the vein, the thrombus (blood clot) is almost always very firmly adherent to the vessel walls so that there is essentially no danger of its breaking off and going to the lungs. In these cases as well as in chronic phlebitis we have effectively used alternating hot and cold whirlpool treatments: 5 minutes in the hot water, 30 seconds to one minute for the cold. Repeat 3-5 times. Use the treatment once or twice a day until symptoms subside.

Pleurisy

Pleurisy is an inflammation of the membranes that cover the lungs and line the chest cavity. During respiration, the irritated surfaces rub across each other painfully. As in bronchitis, place the patient in a chest heating compress, then a long sleeve shirt or sweater to completely cover the arms. Blood must be equally distributed between the trunk and extremities. Then place a double fomentation pack crosswise over the chest and well down both sides under the arms. Cover with plastic to retain heat for 20 minutes. Remove, and place a second pack (no cold between) for 20 minutes, then a third. Finish with a warm shower, a warm friction sponge bath, or an alcohol rub. Use a heating compress to the chest at night.

One should be aware that in the elderly pleurisy is sometimes associated with serious underlying disorders such as pneumonia, pulmonary embolism, tuberculosis, or cancer. Only rarely are these present in the young. If the patient does not respond rapidly to the measures described, a search for other disorders is mandatory.

Pneumonia, Lobar

The pneumococcus is usually the infecting organism. Legionnaire's disease may also give lobar pneumonia. Temperatures may run as high as 105° to 106°. Chilling is one of the most significant factors in lowering body defenses and producing the pneumonia. Three successive stages of pneumonia are recognized including congestion, exudation of blood and blood products into the air sacs, with subsequent consolidation caused by the coagulation of the blood products. Rational treatment should be directed toward relieving the congestion, and producing fluxion of the area to prevent consolidation, or facilitate the removal of consolidated material already formed.

Combine the treatment of a hot foot bath with fomentations to the chest, cold to the head and a fomentation to the spine, followed by cold mitten friction, repeated once or twice daily. Persistently, carefully and properly done, this is an effective method of treatment for lobar pneumonia.[146]

With the patient lying in bed, give a hot foot bath, fomentations over the part of the chest in which pain is located, a fomentation beneath the patient, a cold cloth to the forehead. Only the first treatment should be prolonged to the point of profuse sweating. A hot drink may be used to enhance sweating. When profuse sweating has occurred, the feet and skin of the chest are thoroughly reddened, the treatment being then terminated by a cold mitten friction.

The following points are unusually important: (1) The room should be warm but never warmer than about 72° F. and 65° to 68° are better as breathing warm air is not good for the lungs. (2) Avoid chilling any part of the patient during the treatment or at any subsequent time.[146] It is especially important to avoid the slightest or most brief chilling of the feet; avoid even touching the bare feet to a cold floor. (3) Applications must be quite hot. (4) Fomentations should be large and thick, but should not be a heavy weight on the patient that will inhibit free breathing. (5) Changes should be made very quickly without exposure. (6) Cold mitten friction should be energetic, brisk, and to only one small part of the body at a time, the hot applications being removed only as that part of the body is reached during the cold mitten friction at the end. (7) Remember to dry the skin thoroughly, and handle sweating by repeated drying of the skin. Sweating always endangers the patient to chilling and should be dealt with promptly. It is worthy of repeating that no patch of skin or any part of the body be allowed to become chilled in pneumonia. (8) Use an assistant to support the patient during any part of the treatment requiring physical exertion beyond the strength of the patient.

The daily program should include one full treatment in the morning. No special attempt should be made to cause perspiration after the first treatment, especially if the patient is very weak, but the reaction of redness should be expected and sought for. Subsequent treatments should be quite hot, but not prolonged beyond the comfortable endurance of the patient. Each hot treatment should be concluded with a cold mitten friction. If the patient is very ill, the full treatment should be repeated in the late afternoon. If the patient is not very ill, the afternoon treatment may include only a hot foot bath, fomentations to the upper chest for cough, a massage or an enema if needed. Do not allow the development of constipation or gas as irritating intestinal gases are excreted via the lungs. Inhalations of medicated steam are often helpful. Delirium may occur. Cold compresses to the head are helpful in delirium. Dehydration should be studiously avoided by urging water drinking many times daily. Keep a record of intake and output of fluids. Remember that around two quarts of fluid are ordinarily needed by a healthy person, and a person with a fever or receiving sweating treatments will need more. Count on 2 quarts plus an equal quantity for all that is lost in urine and vomitus. Chapped lips indicate dehydration. Prevent severe cracking from fever blisters by using vaseline. Hot water to drink may be better than cold if there are abdominal complaints. All treatments should be given with attention to avoiding fatigue. Do not discontinue treatments too soon; they should be continued at least two or three days after the fever has subsided, though tapered in length and frequency.

Poliomyelitis

It is urgent to begin treatments immediately when symptoms appear. The patient should be given a full-body pack twice a day. If there is pain between treatments, use a heavy spinal fomentation for thirty minutes.

This extra treatment will relieve pain and reinforce the regular treatments.

Pregnancy Problems

A. Nausea and vomiting of pregnancy—The heating trunk pack with a hot water bottle to the upper abdomen was once called "an almost never failing remedy." It is also indicated in persistent vomiting from other causes. Apply for 20 minutes before the scheduled meal and leave it on for a full three and a half hours after a meal. This treatment has a higher effectiveness than any other form of treatment. It should be used for two meals of the day.
B. Uterine atony during labor—Cold applications over the lower abdomen, short cold applications to the breasts, and alternating hot and cold applications applied to the breasts and lower abdomen will often stimulate uterine contractions in arrested labor.

Prostatitis

Along with hydrotherapy, essential to recovery is an improved body chemistry achieved through diet correction, and exclusion of harmful substances which irritate the genitourinary tract. These include tobacco, caffeine, alcohol, chocolate, vinegar, spices, synthetic food additives, and drugs.

The hot sitz bath, with or without an alternating cold sitz, is the mainstay of hydrotherapeutic measures for the prostate. The hot foot bath should be very hot—a few degrees hotter than the sitz. The hot foot bath may be used alone as a good treatment. It increases the flow of blood to the prostate and its neighboring structures. Use also a lower-half body pack, and lay a thick hot pack across the lower abdomen and pubic area for 15 minutes. Remove, rub the red area vigorously with a cold sponge, and replace with a fresh hot pack. Repeat four times. Finish the treatment with a cool shower, cold mitten friction, or sponge bath. A small, hot, retention enema, with water temperature at 108° to 112° is quite helpful. For urinary retention or inability to void, use a very hot pack to the spine for 20 minutes.

Pyelonephritis

This condition is often serious and accompanied by high fever—104° to 105°— and pain and tenderness in the back just above the waist. Treat the disease diligently with a hot fomentation over the back as in kidney stone (see Stones). Make the applications 45 minutes long and repeat every 3 to 4 hours until the fever drops below

100°. These patients may become very sick, with prostration and high fevers. Give plenty of fluids, but do not overload the sick kidney. Give the supportive measures used for other inflammations and infections.

Rheumatic Fever

The cold bath or cold pack is considered by some to be the best hydrotherapeutic measure for rheumatic fever.[147] Others, however, use the artificial fever. Dunn and Simmons commented on 15 cases of acute rheumatic fever treated by fever therapy, three of which were complicated by chorea. Fourteen patients became symptom-free. Three had relapses and one showed moderate improvement although there were still some rheumatic manifestations three months after completion of 48 hours of fever treatments between 103° and 105° F. Fever therapy promptly reduced the symptomatic activity of rheumatic fever and the leukocyte counts and sedimentation rates became normal in the 14 patients who responded.[148]

Simmons points out that of nine cases of acute rheumatic fever with active endocarditis, six became inactive in an average of 24 days, following an average of five fever treatments.[149][150]

Shingles (Herpes Zoster)

Shingles, a virus infection of the posterior horns of the spinal column and the sensory nerves branching from it, produces severe nerve inflammation in persons who have had chickenpox in earlier life. In adults, shingles can be followed by pain in the area called "postherpetic neuralgia," which can last for weeks, months, or for life. Treatment with the natural remedies in the early stages must not be neglected.

Immediately upon diagnosis put the patient into a full-body pack or a heated tub or whirlpool to induce fever of 102° daily for three to five days or until the skin eruptions dry up. An early, mild case may subside with three treatments. An advanced, severe case will require more. The treatments often have been completely curative, even when they are not begun until three weeks or more after the onset of the disease. Some cases will require also regular massage, charcoal poultices, diet restricted in fats and sugars, and general supportive measures.

Sprains, Ankle

As soon as possible after the accident, seat the patient in a chair in front of two deep pails of water—a hot one maintained at 110° to 120°, and the other well iced.

Put the injured foot into the hot water for three minutes, then into the ice water for one-half minute. Repeat ten times, or until the pain and swelling are gone, which may require an hour or two. Dry the foot thoroughly, and apply a two inch adhesive tape in a figure of eight ankle bandage support. Do not bandage the entire circumference of the extremity as that may cause swelling. Reinforce with extra strips of adhesive if needed. (See illustration) Keep the patient's weight off the foot for about 24 hours. Do not walk on it until it is healed; use crutches.

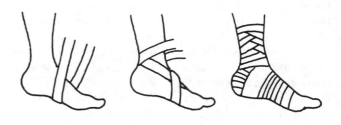

Stroke

Use hot foot or leg baths with ice cravat, ice cap or cold compress to the entire face and scalp, or prolonged tepid baths with water temperature down as low as 90°. The objective is to lower the body temperature as much as possible without inducing shivering.[151] See also Intracranial Bleeding.

Syphilis

Fever therapy will rapidly heal the primary chancre, but must be prolonged in order to prevent secondary syphilis from occurring. To treat a syphilitic interstitial keratosis or iridocyclitis (or gonorrheal conjunctivitis), use fever treatment.[144] See also the section on gonorrhea.

Fever treatments in three hour sessions for syphilis were adopted in 1937, and have been generally used since then. Prior to that, five hour sessions up to 105° and 106° rectally at weekly intervals for a total of up to 50 hours were the usual course, the average patient receiving 36 hours of fever. Since 1937, about 25 hours of therapy have been the average. The three-hour sessions can be given at weekly or semi-weekly intervals to ambulatory patients and three times weekly to those under constant surveillance. The first treatment is about one hour at 102° to 103° rectally, the next at 103° to 104°, the third at 104° to 105°, and the remainder 105° to 106°. The length of time is gradually increased until the patient is able to take three hours of fever at 105° to 106°.

In treating syphilis it is well to be aware of an unusual, always puzzling occurrence, the Jarisch-Herxheimer reaction. It is generally a single episode of headache, flushing, sweating with fever which may go to 104°, starting some two to twelve hours after beginning any drug treatment for syphilis. It occurs in approximately 50% of cases of early syphilis after the first dose of penicillin. It was first observed after mercury inunctions, and was seen also after bismuth and arsenic. Most of the reactions last 24 hours or less.[153] We have no information that it occurs with hydrotherapy, but it is well to remember that the reaction has been reported in the course of treating syphilis with several other methods of treatment.

Tetanus

Fever therapy has been successfully used by others for chronic tetanus.[154] We believe it would be effective in active tetanus as well, but we have not had a case. The important thing is to prevent the infection in very traumatic wounds and deep puncture wounds that allow the anaerobic (without air) growth of the Claustridium germ that causes tetanus. We begin the treatment of the wound at its occurrence, keeping it open to the air if possible, giving excellent cleansing, alternating hot and cold baths, total body massage, poultices, and the proper use of charcoal both internally and externally. With this treatment for wounds we believe the growth of Claustridium is discouraged.

Typhoid

While the major diagnostic features of typhoid may be high fever with a slow pulse, and diarrhea, the toxic effects of the germ fall mainly on the cardiovascular, nervous and renal systems. Copious quantities of water and other fluids should be taken to assist the kidneys to keep the urine dilute. Small retention enemas may be useful for increasing the total fluids absorbed by the patient. If the patient has uncontrollable diarrhea or dysentery (bloody diarrhea), oral fluids, subcutaneous, or intravenous fluids may be the most favorable routes (see Fluid Administration). When the disease is epidemic, in untreated cases the mortality of typhoid varies from 20 to 40%. With all forms of hydrotherapy, the mortality is not over 7.5%, and may be as low as 1%, about the same or better than with antibiotic therapy, and without the risks.

Thirty-three cases of typhoid admitted to one hospital before hydrotherapy was introduced showed a mortality rate of 24.2%, while in 25 cases treated with hydrotherapy it was 6.6%. Another series showed only 2 deaths in 100 consecutive cases, another of 7.6% in 38 cases.[155] With the improvement of understanding of fluid and electrolyte balance, these figures can be expected to be nearly zero now.

The treatments have three objectives: (1) elimination of the invading germs; (2) elimination of the toxins; (3) protection, maintenance, and comfort of the patient. As in all serious illnesses, treatments may need to involve all modalities of simple treatments—diet, massage, herbal remedies, active and passive exercise, charcoal, and water used internally and externally. To promote the most energetic phagocytic activity of white blood cells, food should be given on as nearly regular schedule as possible, two or three small meals daily, containing no free fats or sugars, and composed mainly of fruits and whole grains. The so-called antibacterial "herbals" such as garlic may be used. A most useful adjunct to hydrotherapy, which must not be neglected in serious illness, is massage, used for the relief of the discomforts of fever and prolonged bed rest, to stimulate the circulation, and enhance immune mechanisms. Use charcoal for diarrhea control, adsorption of toxins from the intestinal tract, and encouragement of secretion of toxins from the blood into the bowel.

The most useful remedy is water, given internally in abundance, and used externally as tub baths—hot and cold, foot baths, cold or hot mitten frictions, cool showers or pail pours, etc. Select the treatment based on the major symptoms experienced. Keep the head cool at any time the fever is over 101°.

Gentle cold baths reduce the rate of complications, especially in the respiratory and circulatory tracts. Hemorrhage from the gastrointestinal tract can be treated by brief hot applications to the dorsal and lower lumbar spine at 115° to 120°,[157] rather than hot saline bowel irrigations because of the danger of perforation, which is naturally greater in an infection of the bowel. Use external cold compresses, charcoal poultices or stupes to the abdomen. If diarrhea is frequent, it is desirable to give the charcoal dose after each diarrheic stool.

In the past some have used the Brand Bath, or cold bath, when the fever was above 101°. The cold bath is said to be effective in typhoid, as it not only lowers the temperature by abstracting heat and dilating the surface vessels, but it also aids in the removal of conditions which cause elevated temperature. Nerve impulses are stimulated by a cold bath, vital functions are energized, and oxygenation and metabolism are improved, assisting in the degradation of toxins and elimination of bacteria. We believe, however, that hot baths, in most instances, will be more effective, and certainly more pleasant than the Brand Bath. We include the cold bath for completeness, and for historical interest. Its use has seemed unnecessarily severe to us.

The Brand Bath is a bath at 65° to 70°, the patient being lifted from the bed into the tub as quickly as possible, face and head having been previously cooled by compresses from water at 50°. Immerse the patient to the neck, covering shoulders and knees with towels dipped in the cold water. Wrap the head with towels dipped in the cold water in such a manner that the ends of the towel trail off the back of the head and down the neck, to form a sort of trough.

The patient is rubbed vigorously and constantly upon entering the tub, for 2 to 3 minutes, then sits up for a few seconds while 2 or 3 gallons of water at 50° are poured on his head, and down the towel trough at the back of the neck. The patient again lies back, and is rubbed vigorously for 5 minutes. The water is again poured on the head.

When the patient first enters the bath, he will be gasping and muscles will contract. This unpleasant sensation will be immediately relieved by pouring the cold water on the head. Continue the alternate rubbing and cold water pouring for 10-20 minutes. For infants and elderly, the bath should be shorter. If cyanosis, marked shivering, or teeth chattering occur, remove the patient at once from the water, wrap snugly in a sheet covered by a blanket, put a hot water bottle to the feet, and rub the limbs. Whenever the temperature reaches 101.4° after giving a Brand bath it should be given again. Continue the baths during convalescence to reduce the occurrence of late complications.[157]

Undulant Fever

Employ the same treatment as for shingles, except with a day between treatments, until the symptoms subside—usually five treatments. If after a lapse of time traces of fever recur, repeat the treatment.

Uremia

Uremia results from a failure of kidney function. In acute cases give two treatments daily. Fluids may have to be severely restricted as the kidneys may not be able to put out much water, and the patient will become waterlogged and swollen. Gauge the intake by the amount of urine production, the sweating, and the fluid content of the bowel movements.

Put the patient in a lower-half body pack, and cover the abdomen with a fomentation pack for 15 minutes. Follow with a three minute cold rub to the abdomen and the lower back, turning the patient on one side for the rub. Repeat four times. If necessary, renew the hot pack underneath after the second cold rub. Finish with a shower, or a sponge bath.

Several hours later put the patient into a full-body fomentation, add an abdominal pack, wrap the feet in a fomentation pack, and cover the patient well to cause profuse sweating. Keep the face cool with an electric fan or cold cloths. Check the pulse periodically, and keep it below 120 in a debilitated patient. Continue the pack for 30 minutes. Finish with a bath. Repeat daily until recovery.

Treat uremia also with large charcoal poultices over the abdomen or back each night and four to eight charcoal tablets by mouth four times daily. Give enemas as needed to prevent constipation from the charcoal. A charcoal enema may be helpful in removing toxins. Chronic, progressive uremia indicates more than 90% loss of kidney function, and will require renal dialysis for survival.

Whooping Cough

A danger in whooping cough is exhaustion from violent coughing. Besides the usual measures of good elimination, steam inhalation, light diet, and quiet, the patient will benefit by a daily or twice daily spinal steam pack. It loosens the mucus in the bronchial tubes, allays the irritating cough, intensifies the germ-killing activity of the white blood cells, and relaxes and soothes the patient. A small sip of honey-eucalyptus cough syrup may be given as often as needed. (Stir a drop of eucalyptus oil into a tablespoon of honey.) If ever good hydration is needed, it is in whooping cough. Use every means to increase water drinking, but do not give juices between meals. Various types of hot or cool tea, mint, red clover, lemon grass, or catnip with a twist of lemon, a sprig of rose leaves or geranium petals can all make water more appetizing. Mullein and slippery elm teas are soothing, and have some expectorant effect.

CHAPTER FOURTEEN

Massage

Introduction

Speaking of massage we read in the *Transactions of the American Hospital Association* for 1930, "There is probably no other measure of equal value in the entire armamentarium of medicine which is so inadequately understood and utilized by the profession as a whole."[158] Massage as a physical therapy modality has been relegated to the basement, not because it is ineffectual, but because of being crowded out by machines, appliances, and new techniques. It needs to be restored to its rightful main floor position.

Definitions

There are three essential manipulations: stroking, compression, and percussion. Stroking consists of a gliding movement with a superficial pressure to secure a reflex sedative effect, or deep pressure to reflexively increase venous and lymphatic return.

Stroking:

Effleurage is the principle stroke and is firm but gentle. Effleurage has a definite relaxing effect upon muscles, and should be used in muscle spasm, as in fractures or spastic conditions, pain and myositis. Effleurage has also the effect of sedation. Centripetal effleurage toward the heart hastens the circulation; the lighter rotary or spiral effleurage stimulates the smaller vessels, capillaries and arterioles. Superficial stroking, which is intended to secure reflex effect, must be performed slowly, gently, and rhythmically (10 to 12 strokes a minute).

Compression:

Compression consists of kneading and friction. Compression strokes are designed to improve circulation, hasten the removal of waste products, or break up adhesions or fibrous nodules. It dilates blood vessels; brings relaxation by a direct effect on the muscles; acts as a derivative; and establishes axon reflexes through the spinal cord. It has the effect of relaxing vascular or muscular spasm to relieve pain or discomfort, and promoting the absorption of hemorrhage and exudate by improving blood and lymphatic circulation. Petrissage improves the skin tone. It should develop no friction, but should be a picking up and squeezing of the particular muscular and subcutaneous tissues. In deep friction, the palm is placed against the skin surface, and the skin is rotated without moving the hand over the surface of the skin, so that friction develops in the deeper tissues. Avoid the use of a lubricant in both friction and petrissage, except to soften the hand of the massagist or to oil scaly or dry skin.

Percussion:

Primary percussion consists of cupping, hacking, slapping and tapping, to which some add vibration and shaking. The effects of percussion are on deeper organs such as deeply situated muscles and arteries, the lungs, the adrenals, the kidneys or pancreas. The effects are also quite pronounced on the skin, subcutaneous and muscular tissues, having about the same effect as compression.

There are times when pain must be induced to secure results, such as in stretching adhesions and in the treatment of fibrositis in muscles or subcutaneous tissue, but generally there is no pain or discomfort in massage. Prolonged, heavy percussion may completely anesthetize a tissue through "fatigue" of the nerve endings. For its soothing effect, effleurage should follow all other strokes, even when it has been applied prior to the use of the more vigorous strokes.

Contraindications to Massage

The contraindications for administering massage

usually given in textbooks are as follows: a swelling that might be a malignancy, a deep inflammatory process, certain skin diseases, acute febrile diseases, recent phlebitis and thrombosis, lymphangitis, osteomyelitis, purulent accumulations and severe degrees of hernia.[159] Judiciously used, even in many of these conditions, massage is a great help in the healing process. Massage should generally not be used on the pregnant uterus.[160]

Physiologic Effects

The greatest value of massage is in its action on the circulatory system. Two modes of action can be recognized—mechanical and reflex. The tissues and organs which can be treated most effectively by massage are the skin, eyes, tonsils, sinuses, thyroid, lymph glands, stomach and intestines, and the skeletal muscles.[161] The physiologic effects of massage include changes in blood chemistry, including increased urinary excretion of nitrogen and phosphorus. Several days may elapse before urinary nitrogen returns to the pre-massage level. There is an increased excretion of uric acid. There is reported a 10 to 15% increase in oxygen consumption and carbon dioxide production following either general or abdominal massage, although some investigators have been unable to duplicate this finding. According to a number of investigators a diuresis follows massage.[162] The specific gravity of the urine, however, remains fairly constant, indicating that solids are mobilized and excreted along with the extra water.

The mechanical effects of massage include the movement of lymph fluid, relaxation of sustained muscle contraction and spasm, decrease in venous pressure and secondarily in capillary pressure, and the relief of edema with its collection of metabolites in stagnant tissue fluid. All of the conditions mentioned produce pressure because of their volume, and because of chemical stimulation of nerves producing pain.

Light stroking or friction causes a brief contraction of the capillaries followed by dilatation. Petrissage or percussion causes a dilatation of the deeper blood vessels.

Reflex vascular effects of massage are mediated first through *capillary contraction* as a response of the capillaries to the stroking pressure, followed by *capillary dilatation* on firmer pressure, and finally assisted by dilatation of the arterioles. The latter is due to the local axon reflex mechanisms, not direct stimulation, as is true with the capillaries. With even more intense stimulation such as pinching, a wheal can be achieved, generally considered undesirable. A triple response of massage can therefore be observed: first blanching, then redness, and then wheal formation. All of these reactions are probably mediated by the liberation of a substance by the cells of

the skin and deeper tissues in response to mechanical stimulation. Certainly the wheal forms in response to a chemical substance. The liberated substance is similar to histamine in its direct effect on capillaries, and the indirect effect through the axon reflex to dilate arterioles, and to cause wheal formation from increased capillary permeability.

White blood cells are increased in the blood following several common activities—bathing, exercise, childbirth, during the active process of digestion, and after a massage. In order to be most effective a massage should take about an hour. However, even one moment of massage can do a small amount of good, and often initiates a train of good reactions through feelings of sympathy and kindness. In about half the cases there is a decided increase in hemoglobin after massage. Winternitz found about 15% increase in hemoglobin after hydrotherapy, and apparently some elevation after massage. In one case reported by John Mitchell of Philadelphia there were 4,500,000 red blood cells at the beginning of the massage, and 6,400,000 at the end. The availability of this many extra red blood cells suggests that many cases of anemia are due merely to a lack of activity in the circulating blood, and following a massage, the already matured erythrocytes make their way into the circulation.[163]

A traumatic massage increases the total platelet count at first, but after prolonged trauma the count drops to normal or below, indicating that some of the platelets have become fixed in the tissues.[164] We feel that generally speaking, a massage that causes pain may be injuring tissues.

After exercise, massage is restorative and promotes relaxation. It has been used to reduce muscle tension, relieve swelling, and prevent soreness. In ancient times professional runners were often given massage at night to encourage restful sleep. Massage combined with other treatments can be used profitably in nervous and emotional disorders.[165]

In one study, twenty-five normal persons showed a significant increase in the muscle enzymes serum transaminase, LDH, CPK, and MK when blood was drawn 8 hours after a very heavily done massage of the large striated muscles of both trunk and limbs. MK was elevated to pathologic serum levels, indicating that a risk might be inherent to patients with dermatomyositis treated by vigorous muscle massage.[166]

Other Benefits of Massage

Connective tissue assumes the function of an organ of metabolism. It helps in the regulation of acid-base balance, water content of the body, and osmotic pressure regulation. Of course, it is effective in combating infections, allergies, and inflammation. Connective tissue has the ability to store fat, sugar, water, and other nutrients. By massage, the functions of connective tissue can be enhanced. Definite physiologic changes are accomplished by massage. A definite rise in the temperature has been recorded in the fingertips during the half hour after a total body massage. Secretory functions such as sweating and adrenalin secretion which are under sympathetic control, increase after massage. These reactions enable the body to fight allergies, pain, infections, and degenerative diseases.[167] Massage has been successfully used in many skin disorders; an example is rosacea, a chronic skin disorder.[168]

Massage reduces arterial blood pressure. All of these effects are usually temporary, and do not produce sustained alterations when measured over 24 hours. In some studies, no immediate or delayed effect has been found on basal consumption of oxygen, or pulse rate of normal persons during or after massage.[169] In another study massage of the back resulted in an increase in the activity of the sympathetic nervous system as indicated by measurements of blood pressure, pulse, respiration, skin temperature, oral temperature, and pupil diameter.

Alcohol Absorption from Skin

Absorption of ethyl alcohol, used by some as a massage lubricant, apparently does sometimes occur through the normal intact skin. Two small children were given alcohol rubs lasting eight minutes while they were properly attached to a basal metabolism machine. The machine was for the purpose of excluding the possibility that inhalation of alcohol fumes contributed to the blood level of alcohol. Blood alcohol concentrations reached only the very low level of 0.025 percent. Ethyl alcohol in animal experiments is apparently absorbed by the skin of normal rats much more slowly than essential and volatile oils. In children, both the skin and the lungs may absorb some alcohol. A six month old infant became comatose following a sponge bath using ethyl alcohol. His blood level reached 220 mg. percent.[170] This high level was undoubtedly enhanced by inhalation.

On the other hand, another experiment showed that no alcohol could be detected in any samples of blood of four children between the ages of 7 and 9, and one adult male whose legs were wrapped securely with saturated bandages containing approximately 200 cc. of 95% ethyl alcohol, covered with rubber sheeting, and sealed with adhesive tape. Towels and blankets covered both legs during an experimental period of nine hours in the case of the children, and four hours in the case of the adult. These findings indicate that no appreciable amounts of

alcohol are absorbed through the intact skin.[171] Care must be used to avoid intoxication by alcohol through inhalation in a poorly ventilated room.

We once measured blood alcohol levels before and after student massages in six individuals who received massage with alcohol as a lubricant, and six who were given massage under the same circumstances but using mineral oil as a lubricant. We could detect no evidence of alcohol absorption into the blood of the six students who received their massages with alcohol.

Techniques of Massage

Success in dealing with sick persons is determined by a number of small matters. Careful attention to many small details will insure success in the application of the simple remedies. Massage is a simple remedy, but carefulness and thoroughness will be more likely to achieve success than will years of training and experience without these attributes.

Massage does not require some special technique or touch that some people innately have and others lack. Massage increases the number of circulating white and red blood cells and stimulates the immune mechanism independent of its stimulus to the circulation.

Functions of Massage

1. Acts as a tonic to increase the tone of the skin, muscles, tendons or blood vessels in a weak or chronically ill person
2. Sedates or stimulates according to the nature of the application
3. Increases lymphatic and venous circulation
4. Stimulates muscles in atrophy
5. Prevents excessive scar formation
6. Relieves pain and swelling in sprains and fractures
7. Stimulates the activity or tone of the intestines

Names of Massage Strokes

1. Effleurage—light stroking, a stroking movement subdivided into superficial and deep
2. Petrissage—firm stroking, a compression movement consisting of kneading and frictions, both deep and superficial
3. Percussion—gentle beating with the flat side of the fist or edge of the open hand (Often designated as tapotement, including hacking, tapping, clapping, and beating)
4. Touch—the simple placing of the hand to mold over a part

5. Vibration—done with the hand or a mechanical device, with touch or effleurage
6. Joint movements—passively taking a body part through its range of motion
7. Nerve compression—locating a nerve by palpation, then exerting firm pressure
8. Centripetal—a movement toward the center of the body
9. Centrifugal—a movement away from the center of the body

Lubrication

Vegetable oil and mineral oil are equally satisfactory as massage lubricants. Mineral oil is cheaper. It is not absorbed by the skin. Hand lotion and baby oils may be used if necessary. A drop of oil of wintergreen, musk, clove, cinnamon, lemon, or other oils may be added to scent the massage oil. Do not use the same scent continuously over many months or years as it may irritate, or reduce skin resistance to disease.

Some patients prefer powder to oil on their skin, and the wishes of the patient should be honored as far as possible. Talcum powders should be avoided, and starch powders chosen instead, because of the danger of breathing in the talc and causing scarred nodules in the lungs. A good body rub may be given with your hand dipped in water and used to friction the skin, or with a dry or wet mitten or cloth wrapped around the hand to give friction to the skin, as in the cold mitten friction. A dry, bare hand rub may also be effectively given. This rub is usually short, and often follows a simple procedure such as a foot bath. A most satisfactory lubricant is mineral oil mixed with equal portions of alcohol. The bottle should be shaken before use and may be sprinkled through a cork sprinkler on the hands of the massagist.

Preparation of the Patient

Choose a warm, quiet, softly lighted room with a sturdy table. The patient's bed may be used, but is usually too low and too yielding. A mat on the floor may be used. Have the patient undress and cover with a sheet. Have three small linen towels available for covering the breasts, the genital area and the eyes. While one part is being massaged, the remainder of the body should be fully draped. A light blanket may be needed. Talk very little during the massage, but do not hesitate to ask the patient how he feels, to encourage the patient to breathe deeply and to relax. Pour approximately three-fourths teaspoon of oil into your palm at one time. Apply the oil with both palms, using a simple stroking movement which is gentle, definite, and steady. Try to minimize the

number of times that you remove both hands from contact with the patient. In this way, the patient will have no uncertainty as to what you are doing, or where you are. The massage may begin with the back, the hands or the face. Never make the slightest apology to the patient for your lack of skill, but be ready with a light "excuse me" should you bump, scratch, or otherwise hurt the patient or make a loud noise as by dropping something.

A tickling sensation, or extreme sensitivity of the skin may be encountered along the ribs, on the soles of the feet, or over the abdomen due to excessive sensitivity of the nerve endings. Heavy, firm pressure beginning some distance from the ticklish area will often quiet the tickling sensation. Some persons can tolerate the stroke better if their own hand is placed on top of yours while you are making the stroke. With some persons, the sensitive areas must be omitted in the massage.

If you have time for only a ten minute massage, include the back, the feet, and the upper extremities. If time is short, it is usually well to spend most of the time on the back. Try to eliminate trembling, jerking, and unnecessary stops and starts. Changes in either speed or pressure should be gradual.

When possible, use your weight rather than your hand and arm muscles to apply pressure. You do not need to be physically powerful to do massage. If you find that you experience fatigue or backache after giving a massage, pay attention to how you are standing during the massage. A stance to try is as follows: feet apart, knees bent and turned outward while keeping the back straight. When you first try it, this stance may feel awkward. Having your feet apart, a couple of feet when necessary, permits you to swing your entire body without putting undue stress on large muscle groups of your back to support your weight. Instead, your weight shifts from one foot to another. Lowering yourself by bending at the knees rather than bending your back forward eliminates the strain and fatigue in your lower back.

Massage Strokes

Introduction

A complete massage takes about 30 to 60 minutes. You should yourself do all the lifting or positioning of the part you are massaging. Give the instruction to relax as much as possible. Your inexperience or clumsiness is not likely to be sensed even by a patient who has had many rubs before. Do not call the slightest attention to your lack of experience or inadequate training, or the contrary—how many persons you have treated.

1. Head and Neck

Stand at the head of the table or to the side of the bed. You may use a special non-oily facial lotion on the face to minimize getting the hair oily.

A. Before applying lotion, cover the forehead with the heels of your hands, letting the fingers extend down the temples. Gently rotate the hands. Fig. 1.

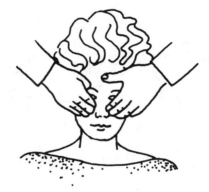

1.

B. Using your thumbs, start at the center of the forehead, stroking both thumbs at once in either direction outward. Press only moderately. Immediately pick up your thumbs, return to the center of the forehead, and work down a second strip, ending in a small circle on the temple. Figs. 2 and 3.

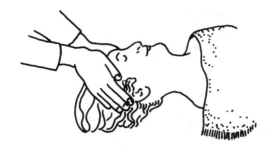

2.

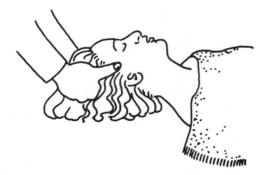

3.

C. Massage the bony rims of the eye sockets with your thumbs, while the fingers rest gently over the face.

Use deep friction for the sinuses, but without stretching the skin of the face.

D. Lightly massage the eyes with your thumbs straight across the closed eyelids, using a minimum of pressure. Repeat three times, moving thumbs in the same direction. Fig. 4.

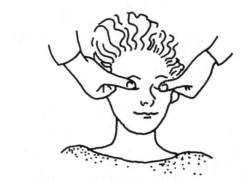

4.

E. Starting just beside the nose, massage the fleshy parts of the cheeks, drawing the tips of the fingers in a path around the lower edge of the cheek bones toward the ears and back up to the temples for a circle. Work the muscles by making tiny circles with your finger tips with only moderate pressure. Fig. 5.

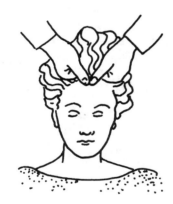

5.

F. Stroke around the ears with the tips of your fingers several times, moving the ear gently and smoothly. End the massage of the ear by lightly pinching the outer edge of the ear between the thumb and forefinger while gently rotating your thumb and forefinger. Fig. 6.

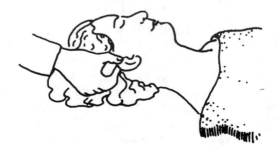

6.

G. Place your left hand under the patient's head, and with your right hand squeeze the muscles in the back of the neck, gently rotating the hands as you squeeze. Change hands, and use the same motion with the opposite hand. Be fairly gentle here, as many people have sore necks.

H. Reposition yourself, this time at the side of the patient, and slip your unlubricated fingertips into the hair, allowing the fingers to spread out to cover the entire scalp, if possible. With a gentle, rotary action, massage the entire scalp for a few seconds.

2.   Chest and Abdomen

A. Main stroke. Stand above the patient's head and place your hands with palms down in the middle of the chest. Be careful that you are high enough above the patient that your clothing does not touch the patient's hair or face, or your position must be at the side of the patient. Glide both hands forward, pressing firmly on the chest, and more lightly on the abdomen, separating the hands at mid-abdomen and moving downward to the sides, then drawing the hands back toward the starting point in a circle above the breasts, avoiding them. Repeat this major stroke six to eight times. Fig. 7.

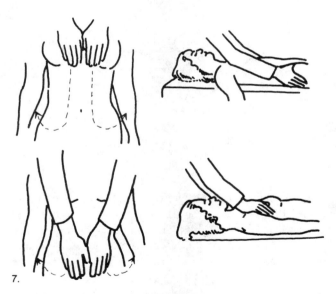
7.

B. "Fulling." Standing at the side of the patient, reach directly across to the far side of the trunk, beginning where fingertips touch the table, firmly draw each hand alternately straight up from the table, across the midline. With each stroke, begin the stroke with one hand just before the other is about to finish, so that there is no break between strokes. Start at the pelvis, just above the thigh, and work your way slowly up to the armpits and then back again. Each stroke should cover a little less than the width of one hand. Exchange sides and repeat. Fig. 8 and 9.

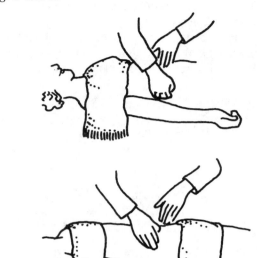
8.

9.

C. Stand at the right side. Support the knees in the slightly bent position by bolsters to relax the abdominal muscles. Beginning in the right lower quadrant with the fingers of your right hand, apply deep, but gentle pressure in full circles about the size of an orange over the outline of the colon, inching along from the cecum up the ascending colon, across the transverse and down the descending colon. Repeat about six times. Fig. 10.

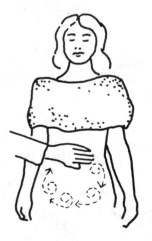
10.

3.   The Hand and Arm

A. Grasp the hand so that your fingers are on the back of the hands. Press into the palm with your thumbs moving them in small circles. Work downward, eventually ending with the fingers. Fig. 11.

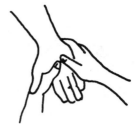

11.

B. Beginning with the palms, start a kneading and squeezing stroke in a hand-over-hand fashion, moving upward on the forearm and ending at the shoulder, returning by stroking the arm downward. Repeat this stroke two or three times. Figs. 12 and 13.

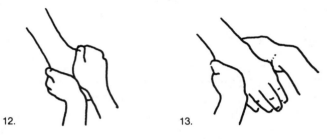

12.   13.

C. Raise the arm, ring the wrist with your thumb and fingers, and massage toward the heart, and return to the original position with a gentle stroke. Repeat several times. Fig. 14.

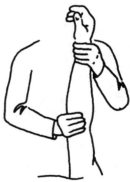

14.

D. Range of motion. Gently work the joints of the upper extremity in their range of motion, beginning with the fingers, proceeding to the wrist, the elbow, and the shoulder. Repeat the entire procedure for the hand and arm on the opposite side. Fig. 15.

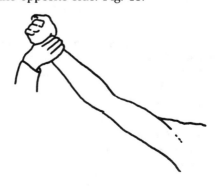

15.

4. Feet

A. Separate the feet several inches, and grasp the foot as you did the hand, and work the soles and tops of the feet at the same time, the thumbs separating and massaging the muscles on the top of the foot while the fingertips are separating and massaging the tissues on the opposite side of the foot. Fig. 16.

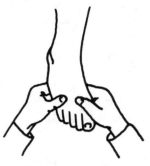

16.

B. To massage the heel, gently lift the foot from the table with the left hand, and work the heel by pressing the thumbs and fingertips into the tissues and firmly rotating, beginning at one portion of the heel, and gradually working each part. Fig. 17.

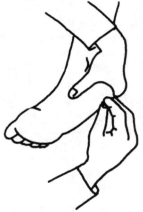

17.

C. Next, squeeze the foot just as you did the hand, in a hand-over-hand motion, beginning at the base of the toes and ending at the knee. Fig. 18.

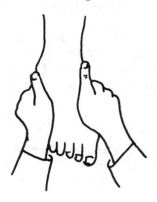

18.

D. Using some force, bend the foot in each direction possible—hands positioned as in A above, attempting to roll the foot into a cylinder. Bend the toes, then the whole foot down, then the whole foot upward to stretch the Achilles tendon.

5. Front of the Leg and Thigh

A. Long stroke. Standing at the foot of the table, with the lubricated hands at the ankle, cupped across the top of the leg, fingers pointing inward in opposite directions, glide both hands from the ankle steadily up the leg, using moderate pressure from your own shoulders, moving more lightly across the knees, and again firmly onto the thigh, letting the hands separate above midthigh, beginning a circle downward along the sides to return to the ankle. Repeat five or six times. Fig. 19.

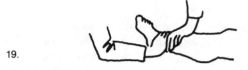

19.

B. Petrissage. This stroke is done on the top of the thigh and is a combination of a slap, a pinch, and a knead. It is done by rapidly alternating the action of the two hands as follows: slap the slightly cupped hand onto the thigh and grasp the tissue in the cupped hand, pinching it fairly firmly, lifting up slightly, and releasing the tissue quickly. As the first hand is releasing the tissue, the opposite hand is beginning the slap, pinch, lift and release. The stroke is done rapidly about two per second, moving from the knee to the pelvis and back again. Repeat for the opposite thigh.

6. Back of the Leg

A. Have the patient lie on the stomach, spread oil over one leg, thigh, buttock and hip.

B. Place the patient's feet a foot or so apart. Mold the hands across the back of the ankle, with the fingertips pointing in opposite directions. Firmly move both hands up the leg, separate hands at the top of the thigh similarly as on the front of the leg, moving the outside hand in a wide arc over the top of the hip, tracing the curve of the hip bone in a circle along the front of the hip, moving back down the side toward the foot. At the same time move the left hand in a smaller arc down the inside of the thigh and back to the ankle. Repeat this stroke three or more times. Fig. 20.

C. Wringing. Cup both hands side by side, thumbs together, grasping the base of the patient's calf. Twist the left hand away from you and around the leg at the same

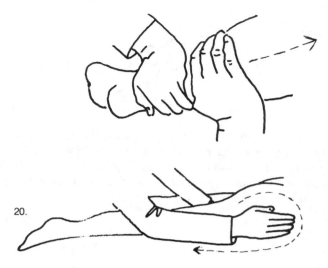

20.

time you twist your right hand toward you, and around the leg, resembling an "Indian burn." Reverse directions, working gradually up the length of the leg. The hand movement, though light in pressure, should be as fast and vigorous as possible without sacrificing definiteness. Keep the thumbs always brushing against each other. Fig. 21.

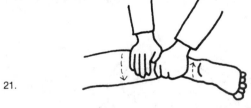

21.

D. Stripping. Encircle the leg and slowly glide up the leg, squeezing gently with the palms and thumbs alike, ending at the knee and returning to the ankle at the same slow pace, but without pressure. Repeat the stroke for the thigh. Fig. 22.

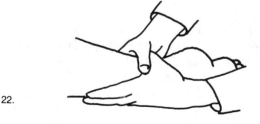

22.

E. Raking. This is a good stroke for stimulation anywhere, but especially on the thigh and back. Holding each hand with the fingers spread slightly apart and curved, stiffen the fingers, so that hand looks somewhat like a claw. Move down the length of the thigh, with short raking, alternating strokes, beginning at the top of the thigh or on the buttock, work rapidly and firmly, each stroke about 6 inches long, ending at the ankle. Fig. 23.

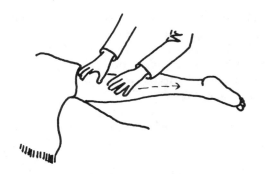

23.

F. Finish the leg by flexing it onto the buttock, gently pushing it into extreme flexion, bouncing it several times in this position.

7. Buttocks

A. Kneading. Lift the flesh, squeeze, knead rhythmically, both hands constantly touching the skin, but alternating hands for the squeeze. Massage one buttock thoroughly from waist to thigh, and then move on to the other. Fig. 24.

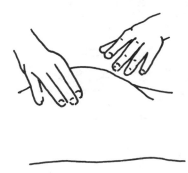

24.

B. With the fingertips, knuckles, or heel of one hand, lightly probe the flesh about an inch to the side of the center of one buttock. Locate a slight indentation between two large muscles, the Gluteus medius and the Gluteus maximus. Press the heel of the hand or a knuckle into the indentation. Vibrate the hand as fast as practicable for about ten seconds, then move to another part of the buttock in a circle, or in vertical lines. Repeat for the opposite side. Fig. 25.

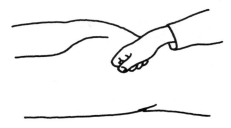

25.

8. The Back

A. Spend more time on the back than on any other part. Spread oil very lightly over the back, shoulders, and sides of the trunk.

B. Main stroke. Stand at the head or side of the table. Beginning at the top or bottom of the spine, glide hands along the entire length of the back, using firm pressure, and leaning into the stroke with your own weight. Separate the hands at the end of the spine, moving toward the sides and returning to the starting position by pulling both hands along the sides of the trunk, exerting moderate pressure. Repeat the stroke several times.

C. Place the right hand on the midline of the patient's spine, heel of your hand at the lower end of the spine, fingers pointing toward the head. Add extra pressure by placing your left hand on top of your right. Slowly glide the hands straight up the spine, with moderate and steady pressure. At the top of the back, return the stroke at the same speed, but with the forefinger and middle finger pressing into the furrows that lie on either side of the spine, lifting the heel of the hand out of contact with the patient. Use as much pressure on your fingertips as possible. Repeat this stroke several times. Figs. 26 to 28.

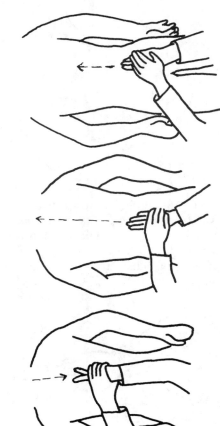

26.

27.

28.

D. Upper back. Knead the trapezius muscles by squeezing with the thumbs, and fingers. Fig. 29.

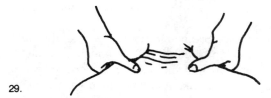

29.

E. Shoulder blades. Place the patient's right hand, palm up, in the middle of his back. Lift his shoulder an inch or two from the table, and slide your right forearm in such a manner that, as you are standing at the head of the table, the patient's shoulder will rest in the crook of your right elbow, your right hand grasping the forearm immediately below his elbow. In this position the shoulder blade is raised, and the fingers of your left hand can be run around the elevated scapula with firm pressure. Repeat several times. Cupping the hand over the shoulder blade, fingers apart, move the skin over the shoulder blade in wide circles, several times to the right and then to the left. Repeat for the left side. Fig. 30.

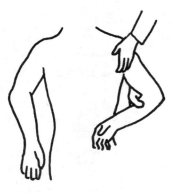

30.

F. Friction. Pull one hand toward you as you push the other away from you, beginning at the top, and moving down the entire length of the spine and back again. Generate as much friction on the skin as possible, keeping the hands moving constantly and rapidly. Fig. 31.

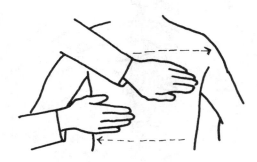

31.

G. Place two of your fingers, or your thumbs, one on each side of the spine, beginning at the neck, and, proceeding the entire length of the spine. Massage in about one inch circles between the spinous processes to stimulate the large nerve trunks as they come out from between the vertebrae. Fig. 32.

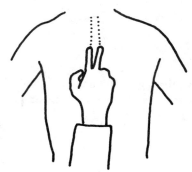

32.

H. Hacking. Hold your hands palms facing together and fingers loosely apart. Drum the outer edges of your hands very lightly and rapidly against the fleshy parts of the back, beginning at the shoulders and going up and down the spine once or twice. Fig. 33.

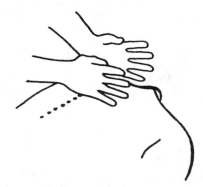

33.

I. Feather stroke. Using both hands at once, stroke straight down the back from neck to buttocks, using the fingertips only, as lightly as possible to continue to maintain contact with the skin. Fig. 34, 35.

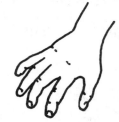

34.

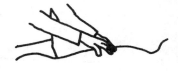

35.

Special Massages

1. Sprains

A. Heat should precede the massage for sprains.

B. Use soothing effleurage to the sprained area, interrupted with petrissage to the more distant unaffected parts of the sprained limb.

C. By the third or fourth day, the petrissage can be given nearer to the sprained area.

D. On the sixth or seventh day the sprained limb is usually supported by strappings or bandages and permitted to be used.

2. Fractures

There is an accumulation of tissue fluids and products of injury that accumulate at the site of the fracture. The application of a cast impedes the removal of this debris, but massage rapidly removes these materials by restoring the local lymphatic and circulatory drainage, increasing the vitality of the tissues and hastening repair.

Six to eight weeks are required to heal a fracture of the leg when treating by the conventional methods of casting for immobilization. Even after these 6-8 weeks the leg is stiff, thin and weak, and shows edema of the skin reflecting the poor nutrition of the soft tissues. When massage and passive exercise are used, and the broken leg is treated without casting, the bone heals in one-third the usual time and the complications of prolonged immobilization are avoided.

Surgeons who have used it say that the correct repair of the bone fracture is not endangered by this procedure provided the cases are selected with care, and those cases rejected for this type of treatment if they show the following features: (1) an extreme tendency for the broken ends to get out of correct position; (2) over-riding of the broken bone ends; and (3) bone fragments or chips in such a position or of such a shape as to easily work through the skin and compound the fracture.

The broken bone should be reduced, that is, the broken ends must be replaced by pulling on the leg in such a way as to put the bone back in its natural position. Then the leg should be securely splinted for several days until there is no deformity or displacement when manual support is substituted for the splint, and there is no pain with the passive motion, perhaps from 4 to 14 days. Daily massage for 15 to 20 minutes and passive motion of the leg is begun when the splints are removed. Some surgeons keep the leg splinted between the daily treatments, but others do not. Patients are able to walk with crutch or cane in an average of 14 days. The total treatment averages 24 days.

To be properly cautious, fractures involving the tibia which show deformity of the leg should always be immobilized in plaster-of-paris. Fractures of the fibula alone may be fearlessly treated by massage and passive motion and the patient allowed to walk in two weeks.[172]

In fractures use a light stroking massage, slow, even, steady, and always in the same direction, lengthwise the part, in the direction of venous circulation. Massage does not rub the exudate out of the part by pressure and force, but reflexively rids the part of tissue hemorrhage and exudate by bringing about improved circulatory conditions. Light and very gentle kneading may be used to advantage in fracture cases. Such movements stimulate the intramuscular circulation and improve muscle tone.[173]

A. Begin massage as early as gentle effleurage can be used without producing pain.

B. Petrissage and passive and active joint movements are usually not used until there is some union of the bone ends.

C. Active and passive movements of the joints on each side of the fracture area assist in reducing adhesions. The movements and the massage should not be excessively applied, as prolonged treatment causes over-excitation of the muscles with resulting spasm, one of the very things one is trying to allay.[174]

3. Scar Tissue and Contractures

A. Friction and petrissage are the strokes used to loosen scars and contractures.

B. Pain must usually be produced to stretch adhesions.

C. The massage should be preceded by heat.

D. Deep digital friction, alternating with effleurage, is the most effective stroke.

E. Joint movements and tendon stretching may be helpful.

4. Varicose Veins

Massage over varicose veins, if it is reasonable and does not include pounding or percussion, can be relaxing and helpful. It is probably not advisable over areas in which varicose ulcers are situated.[175] It is felt by some that phlebitis might be precipitated by the more vigorous types of massage, but the treatment should promote a sense of well-being and relief of congestion and edema, especially if massage is preceded by elevation of the part containing the varicose veins.

5. Tonsillar Massage

A massage of the tonsils is sometimes advocated to increase the general resistance, or to enhance the ability of the tonsils to fight infection either in themselves, or elsewhere in the body. Tonsils are a natural depot of lymphocytes. In chronically enlarged tonsils, the lymphocyte level may be low because of an increase in other cell types that displace the lymphocytes. Massage can increase both the flow of blood in the tonsils and the chemotactic substances of the tissues to draw in more leukocytes. The leukocytes in the circulating blood are also increased by massage.[176] In health there are large numbers of mature lymphocytes that are out of the moving current of the blood. Even those in the blood loiter and delay at certain points in their travels. Studies show that a great number of cells may be brought rapidly into the circulation by massage. It would seem wise to massage the large lymphoid deposits such as tonsils, appendix, and lymph nodes in the groin, armpits, neck, abdomen, and elsewhere, as a general measure for fighting various fevers and infections.

6. Gynecologic Massage

The use of massage in gynecology has assisted in avoiding operations and preserving the generative organs by conservative treatment. The effect of uterine massage is to bring about a healthier state of circulation and to impart tonus to the various structures. Massage is indicated in all chronic inflammatory states as well as in retroversion of the uterus, relaxed ligaments, pelvic exudations, and adhesions. It may be used in cervicitis, cervical polyps, and nonspecific discharges.

The patient should be positioned on her back, with the legs drawn up. A correct diagnosis with the exclusion of all acute pus-producing disorders such as acute pyosalpingitis, and recent ovarian abscesses should be made, as massage in these conditions might cause a spread of the infection.

In gynecologic kneading, the diseased parts are taken between the first three fingers of the inner hand held within the vagina, and the palm of the outer hand placed on the abdomen. The parts are rubbed, pressed, squeezed, and kneaded in such a firm, gentle manner that the patient will not object to having the procedure repeated. The fingers in the vagina are used mainly as a point of support while the external hand manipulates the parts. The massage should not exceed five minutes in length for the first few massages, but later increased to ten or fifteen minutes. In chronic salpingitis the oral temperature should be taken periodically after the massage to make certain that an infection has not flared up.

The second type of gynecologic massage is pressure with stroking. The inner hand fixes the part, the outer hand presses and strokes with moderate force not letting the parts slip back, but gently allowing them to slide

along under constant equal pressure. This is repeated eight or ten times at first, increasing to 20 times at subsequent treatments. The direction to stroke is usually from the fundus of the uterus toward the large vessels on either side or vice versa if the uterus is to be included in the massage. This massage is helpful where there are adhesions around the adnexal tissues.

The third type of gynecologic massage is lifting or stretching. It is similar to the second procedure, but instead of allowing the parts to slide between the two hands, the parts are lifted or moved to the point of discomfort then relaxed while maintaining the grasp. Repeat the stretching 8 to 10 times.

The objectives of massage are to accelerate the absorption of inflammatory exudates or deposits, to stretch and loosen scars, and to stimulate circulation and restore normal elasticity and tone. It is useful in many pelvic exudations and hemorrhagic infiltrations, retroversion and prolapse.[177]

7. Pain Control with Massage

As a modality to control pain, massage is without a peer. In fact, to rub a painful spot is almost reflexive or instinctive in both man and animal. Massage tends to break the cycle of pain which consists of sustained reflex muscle contraction, leading to deep pain and eventually to more reflex contraction. This cycle leads to reflexive sustained muscle contraction with decreased circulation from pressure on vessels and subsequent ischemic pain. The principle of counterirritation as a treatment for pain, inflammation and infection is based on cutaneovisceral reflexes. If pain occurs in an internal organ, there is often a reduced blood supply in the organ or tissues, and the accumulation of chemical wastes, the circulation being inadequate to take the toxins away. The pain is alleviated merely by altering the circulation. Massage improves the circulation through effects on proprioceptive receptors of the skin and underlying tissues.

Because of the anatomical distribution of various types of nerves, stimulation of the skin sends afferent impulses *to* the central nervous system, and axon reflex impulses that operate in an arc to and *from* the spinal cord to act on the arterioles. Therefore, both central and peripheral influences mediate the pain-relieving effects of massage. There are probably also pressure sensitive nerve fibers intermingled among the nerves of the blood vessels of both the skin and deep organs which bring about a fall in blood pressure when they are stimulated, through vasodilatation of the splanchnic region.

The psychological aspects of massage are quite important. Sensory input transmitted through the larger and very efficient myelinated nerve fibers which mediate touch, pressure, and proprioception, can mask sensory impulses arriving over the smaller, and less efficient nerve fibers which mediate sustained painful perceptions. The nerve stimulation from the massage simply arrives at the brain centers before and in larger degree than from the pain fibers. Certainly, the reticular formation of the brain can produce inhibition of sensory impulses as they arrive at receiving nuclei in the central nervous system—yet another way the brain can handle pain.

It has been shown that a cat producing a certain size action potential in the cochlear nucleus from constant clicking sounds will suddenly decrease the action potential size, if her attention is directed off the constant clicking sounds by the introduction of a mouse into her cage. By analogy, one could say that the confidence a patient has in the treatment or in the helper can set up a pattern of inhibition and selective stimulation in the forebrain that influences profoundly any painful impulses. Therefore, compassion and kindness become important therapeutic weapons for the relief of pain.[178] These therapeutic weapons are to be distinguished from the generally unprofitable impulses of sentimentalism and coddling which have no place in the treatment of the sick.

8. Abdominal Massage, and Procedures for Constipation

A. Deep breathing exercises. Take a full inspiration and hold for 20 counts, exhale fully and hold to the count of ten. Repeat 20 to 40 times. Do the exercise 3 times daily while driving or working.

B. The Mosher exercise: Lie on the back on a pad on the floor. Three positions are assumed one after another, continuing for one to three minutes. The positions are as follows: (1) Protrude the abdomen as high above plane as possible and hold for several seconds; (2) Relax the abdominal muscles and assume an "on plane" position; (3) Contract abdominal muscles to "hold in" the abdomen for several seconds; (4) Relax and return to the "on plane" position. Repeat for about 3 minutes.

C. Reflex effleurage: A direct mechanical movement of solid contents of the colon or small intestine is seldom possible by massage, although gas is usually moved readily. It is the reflex action that achieves the benefit. Lie on the back and gently massage the colon. Begin with the fingers of the left hand over the cecum in the right lower abdominal quadrant. Make circular massaging movements, then proceed up the colon a bit for the second series of circular movements. Follow the outline of the colon up and around the hepatic flexure. Change hands smoothly, and continue around the splenic flexure, descending colon, sigmoid and rectum. Repeat eight to ten times.

D. Gentle percussion to colon, tapping, spatting, slapping.

E. Gentle digital kneading of colon, four times as a minimum and up to 10-20 minutes duration.[179]

F. Deep vibration of the colon also may be combined with reflex effleurage. An effective conclusion of the abdominal massage is the "Erschiittering." Place the right hand on the umbilicus, fingers spread and in firm skin contact, and exert a little pressure on the abdomen, the patient completely relaxed. Grasp your right wrist with your left hand and exert evenly a fairly strong trembling movement. Repeat the maneuver in each of the four abdominal quadrants. The patient must be relaxed; therefore it is essential to perform this stroke during the period of exhalation. Instruct the patient to breathe deeply then exhale during the trembling action.[180]

G. Percussion to the lumbar spine.

H. Small cold enema: Use a bulb syringe that will hold about one-half cup of water. Use cold water and only one bulb full. Use after each meal. Gradually the colon will be trained to empty itself after meals if the exercise is continued many weeks on a very regular schedule.

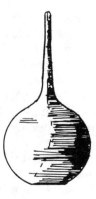

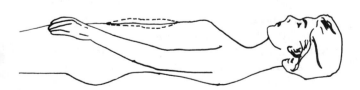

The Mosher Exercise. The abdomen is first protruded, then relaxed, then contracted inward, then relaxed. This exercise massages the internal organs, relieves pain or congestion.

Syringe for the small cold enema. Purchase an "ear syringe" or "infant syringe" from a pharmacy. Use one syringe of cold water for either infant or adult to initiate a bowel movement.

Massage of The Fully Clothed Patient

There is a way to overcome most difficulties that interfere with massage. Occasionally it is not desirable to give a patient a massage directly on the skin surface. The fully clothed patient may be given a massage effectively. Perhaps the room is too cool or drafty, perhaps the patient has a sensation of chilliness even in a warm room, or perhaps the patient's skin is hypersensitive and the touch of the massagist causes a tightening of the muscles or tickling. Sometimes for reasons of modesty it is well to leave the patient fully clothed.

The procedure is essentially the same except that the clothing will impede any gliding motion. Stroking can best be done in the direction of the edge of the clothing to avoid excessive wrinkling. Also, for the patient clad in pajamas, the legs and thighs can be handled by making a reciprocal gliding motion of the hands, one past the other, as one hand glides upward the other is going downward. Such a motion displaces the clothing very little.

A rotary motion with pressure is a good one for the dressed patient, as well as a gripping and pinching of the large muscle groups. The buttocks can be stroked from the bedline on each side to the small of the back, as one stands beside the thighs. The back can be stroked from the shoulders to the waist, as one stands beside the head. The feet may be properly massaged through thick socks used for protection from chilling or to prevent excessive tickling in a very sensitive person. It is often helpful to massage even over thick bandages.

Self-Massage

Introduction

Massage is beneficial, not only because of the enjoyment and relaxation that one gets, but also because of the increase of the circulation, the benefits to be derived from bringing the blood from the interior to the exterior of the body with the reduction of internal congestion, and the addition to the blood of disease-fighting substances by the very helpful macrophages which are stationed in the skin. Through the stimulation to the skin, the production of white blood cells is encouraged, and the addition to the blood of certain antibodies derived from the permanently stationed macrophages occurs.

The best position for a self-massage is lying flat on the back on a carpeted floor, cushions and bolsters used as needed for comfort and support. You may or may not use a massage lotion. The self-massage is at the same time a manipulation of joints, an exercise in flexibility, and an exerciser of shoulder, arm, and back muscles.

1. Grasp the foot with both hands, turn the sole upward into your view, and bury your thumbs into the soles. Massage the various pads of the foot, the pads of the toes, between the toes, and between the bones of the foot. Twist each toe, using a gentle motion. Never over-strain the joints.

2. Raise the knee toward the chest and encircle the leg below the knee as far as you can reach with both hands. Milk upward toward the knee, using a firm and uniform movement.

3. With the thumb and forefinger, pinch the fleshy parts of the calf of the leg, using a kneading and rotary motion combined, to increase the circulation to this part.

4. With the closed fists, pound the thighs from the knee to the groin. Use care to cover all portions, but do not bruise the tissues.

5. Gently bounce the knee toward the chest, trying to get the thigh to lie flat against the abdomen. Repeat all strokes with the opposite extremity.

6. The abdominal massage begins with a gentle rotary motion on the right lower quadrant of the abdomen, rotating the fingers of the right hand in the lower quadrant of the abdomen, moving up an inch or so and repeating, until the right upper quadrant is reached. Continue the gentle rotary movement, inching along across the top of the abdomen until the left side is reached. At that point, begin a series of rotary motions downward toward the left groin. Continue the rotary motion, crossing over the lower portion of the abdomen and proceed with a clockwise spiral until the entire abdomen has been worked over.

7. Using the fingertips of the right hand, massage the muscles of the left chest, using care to get between the ribs quite well. Repeat, using the left hand on the right chest.

8. Use a stiff brush to brush the skin of the neck from the collar bones across the neck, up across the jaws, and cheeks and forehead, up to the hairline. Cover every square inch of skin over the neck, face, and portions of the scalp that are free of hair.

9. Do facial and eye exercises at this point, squeezing the eyelids tightly together and rotating the eyes from side to side, from extreme top to extreme bottom, and in each of the diagonals, right and left. While the facial muscles are contracted, take the fingertips and gently rotate the skin of the face and neck.

10. Rotate the head as far to the right, and then as far to the left as is possible. Put both hands behind the head and bring the head downward toward the chest as far as possible.

11. Do a body twist, turning the shoulders as far as possible in one direction, while turning the hips as far as possible in the other direction.

12. Do a body roll with the arms fully extended overhead. Using the right foot and leg to give a little help, roll two complete turns toward the left. Repeat the movement using the left leg to help, and roll two complete turns back to the right.

Brush Massage

The brush massage is recommended either self-administered or given by a helper. Use a kneading motion over all portions of the body with a stiff brush, keeping the brush in contact with the skin and manipulating it with a circular and creeping movement, varying the speed and pressure of the movements; faster over the large skin areas, and slower and with lighter pressure over the fingers or neck. Use an ordinary firm bristle brush. This type of massage can be used for tics, neurological problems, anxiety states, general physical conditioning, aches and pains, and is especially helpful on the neck and back.

Other Diseases and Massage

Most sicknesses are benefited by massage. Colds, sinusitis, sore throat, and laryngitis all improve with massage. During an upper respiratory tract infection, the nose, cheeks, upper teeth, hard and soft palate should all

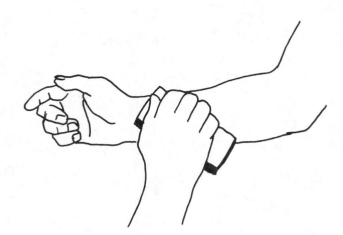

Brush Massage. Using a dry brush with moderately stiff bristles begin with the fingertips and travel slowly up the arm with a circular motion. After the extremities, brush the trunk and the back as well as possible.

be given fingertip massage by stroking and deep rotary pressure, fingers and thumbs used inside the mouth and on the skin. A gentle massage of the abdomen is frequently most helpful in peptic ulcer, gastritis, gas pains, and diarrhea. Skin eruptions may be soothed and assisted by gentle massage. Of course, headaches should always be treated with gentle massage.

CHAPTER FIFTEEN

Charcoal Therapy

Introduction

Many old-fashioned remedies are going out of fashion, not because they are ineffective, but because an art is required for their management, and a sufficient degree of labor required that most people are unwilling to provide. Every private home should have charcoal on hand as a ready antidote for poisoning, and as a cleansing agent in infections and various metabolic disturbances. Orally administered charcoal is effective in preventing many intestinal infections. All studies show that charcoal is harmless when ingested, when inhaled and when it comes in contact with the skin.

Charcoal is without a rival as an agent for cleansing and assisting the healing of the body. The grains of charcoal have many crevices and corners for the adsorption of materials, gases, foreign proteins, body wastes, chemicals and drugs of various kinds making it a powerful assistant to the cleansing apparatus of the body. The total surface area of the sum of the particles in a small cube of charcoal only 2/5th of an inch on each side is one thousand square meters, a field more than thirty-three yards square! The uses of charcoal are almost as universal as those of water, both commercially and medically—and like water it can be freely used as a healing agent. Because charcoal can pack molecules of ammonia gas into its crevices, it can attract 80 quarts of ammonia gas per 1 quart of pulverized charcoal! It may be used internally or externally, and for a range of disorders from bee stings and other venomous bites, to metabolic problems such as jaundice of the newborn, or an allergic reaction to poison ivy.

In 1773, Scheele made an experiment with charcoal in which a gas was trapped in an inverted tube with charcoal, the lower end of the tube submerged in a container of mercury. Most of the gas disappeared as evidenced by a rise of mercury into the tube. As the gas was adsorbed by the charcoal, a vacuum appeared in the tube and sucked the mercury up into the tube. As a demonstration of the effectiveness of charcoal, Bertrand in 1913 survived after swallowing 5 grams of arsenic trioxide mixed with charcoal, and Touery in 1831 survived after swallowing 15 grams of strychnine (ten times the lethal dose) and an equal amount of charcoal before the French Academy of Medicine.[181]

Materials for Making Charcoal

Charcoal can be produced from a number of different materials. Charcoal made from burnt toast is apparently entirely worthless, and the so-called "universal antidote" with glycerin, tea and charcoal is decidedly inferior to plain charcoal, the tannic acid in the tea decreasing the effectiveness of charcoal. Tannic acid as found in many herbs precipitates alkaloids, certain glycosides, and many metals. It interferes with the usefulness of charcoal as an antidote. Willow charcoal, (or any commercial charcoal) is quite effective against bad breath, gas and intestinal disorders.

Charcoals made from vegetable material such as wood and coal, contain about 90% carbon, whereas bone charcoal contains about 11% carbon, 9% calcium carbonate, and 78% calcium phosphate. Bone charcoal is quite effective in decolorizing solutions, and is used widely in the sugar industry for this purpose. Charred coconut or black walnut shells make very good adsorptive material. Such materials as blood, cereals, fruit pits, kelp, corn cobs, rice hulls, distillery wastes and paper mill wastes have all been used to make charcoal. The most common present day charcoals are made from petroleum coke, coals, peat, sawdust, wood char, paper mill wastes, bone and coconut shells.

Activated charcoal is produced from the controlled burning of wood or bone, and is then subjected to the action of an oxidizing gas, such as steam or air, at elevated temperatures. This process enhances the adsorptive power of charcoal by developing an extensive internal network of fine pores in the material. The activation process was invented somewhat after the turn of the 20th century, but charcoal was already recognized as a very useful healing agent, illustrating the efficacy of ordinary charcoal. Nobody has really understood the mechanism by which charcoal works, either from a physical or chemical standpoint.

Charcoal made in the kitchen from such items as bread or burned food is definitely inferior or poor, and may be harmful if used on a regular basis. Wood charcoal is preferred since it does not develop the harmful chemicals (such as methylcholanthrene and benzopyrene) sometimes formed from burned fats.

When making your own charcoal, pieces of charred wood from the fireplace or grill can be used. The ultimate in making your own charcoal begins with a wood fire out-of-doors. After the wood is burning brightly, it should be covered with a large piece of tin, and dirt piled over the tin to make a dome to exclude air. As the heat continues to burn the wood without oxygen, the soft parts of the wood are burned out and the hard parts remain, making a good charcoal. The charred parts of wood should then be pounded to coarse granules in a cloth bag. After it is reduced to chunks ranging in size from small peanuts to rice grains, put the charcoal in a blender and pulverize it to a fine powder, the finest that can be obtained.

The commercial tablets as compared to finely powdered charcoals have been found less effective by about half. In one study [182] humans who took pulverized charcoal were able to prevent absorption of a drug by 73%, whereas those taking the tablets prevented only 48%. A tablet containing 0.44 gm. total material has only 0.33 gm. of charcoal, the remainder of the material representing starch and other substances used to hold the tablets together. Chewing the tablets well before swallowing will increase their effectiveness.

Briquettes used for charbroiling are not safe sources for charcoal for either external or internal use, as various undesirable fillers are used, and chemicals are often applied to the products to insure rapid igniting.

General Features

Charcoal has been used to combat odors in air and water, to remove carbon dioxide from air in submarines, to filter poisons in gas masks, in making medicines, and coloring candy jellybeans and licorice. Charcoal may be powdered and placed in a jar lid on a shelf, in the refrigerator, oven, or a drawer and it will adsorb a variety of odors, including rancid odors. It is useful in removing odors from casts, skin ulcers, and gastrointestinal gas, and as a cigarette filter. Herbicides applied too liberally, or having an inordinately long residual effect, may be

efficiently counteracted by a charcoal spray. It has been used to remove toxins from the blood in kidney and hepatic diseases, taking the charcoal internally, or applying it as a poultice or bath, and for use in an exchange column to perfuse blood.

Except for the occasional finding of irritation of bowel in certain inflammatory states in very sensitive persons, and the prolongation of the transit time sometimes seen, there are no known contraindications to the use of charcoal. Allergies have not been reported. It is inexpensive, harmless and easily applied. It is available readily through commercial channels, or can be made at home.

Care should be used in applying charcoal poultices to freshly broken skin. It is possible to get a tattooing effect if the lesions extend through the skin into the dermis. For such wounds, it is wiser to use comfrey poultices to avoid the possibility of tattooing an area not usually covered by the clothing.

Dosage of Charcoal

One can buy charcoal powder, tablets and capsules. The activated capsules are roughly twice as potent as the tablets. Drug stores or health food stores often carry charcoal. The oral dosage is 1 tablespoon of powder stirred into a glass of water, 4 capsules of activated charcoal, or 8 regular tablets taken in the mid-morning and repeated in the mid-afternoon. Food interferes with its effectiveness. Charcoal probably should not be taken regularly over long periods—years—as some nutrients may be adsorbed. We have seen no problems with its intermittent use for long periods, or with regular use for up to twelve weeks.

Charcoal may be ordered from Yuchi Pines Institute, Rt. 1, Box 273, Seale, Al. 36875.

Because of interference with effective adsorption of toxic materials in the gastrointestinal tract, it is estimated that 10 grams (about 1 tablespoon) of charcoal can adsorb only about three to seven grams of materials, making it necessary to give at least twice the amount of charcoal as the suspected weight of the poison taken.[183]

There has been some discussion as to whether food and partially split derivatives of food, digestive enzymes, and various secretions usually found in the gastrointestinal tract would inhibit adsorption of drugs or poisons by charcoal. It has been found that there is approximately 50% reduction in effectiveness of adsorption with charcoal due to stomach contents, 30% reduction due to bile, and very minor reduction due to duodenal juice. Therefore, when a poison has been ingested, to be on the safe side use approximately eight to ten times the estimated weight of the poison as the dosage of charcoal.

Finely powdered charcoal can get to the surface of toxins better than coarsely powdered charcoal and should be used for the best results.

Charcoal adsorbs poorly mineral acids, alkalis and salts such as NaCl (table salt) and FeSO₄ (iron). There is some advantage in recognizing this particular characteristic of charcoal, since in the area of nutrients, charcoal is a poor adsorbent. Every year children die from poisoning from table salt and iron. Extra large doses of charcoal should be used when these substances have been swallowed.

In combating poisons, the speed with which the charcoal is administered will determine to a certain degree the success. Additionally, the quantity of charcoal is a determinant of success. For venomous bites or poison ivy, immediately wash the area well with soap and water, or flood with a solution of charcoal. After this brief preparation the poultice can be applied.

In cholera, give 2 heaping teaspoons of pulverized charcoal four times daily, and supplement with 1-2½ liters of normal saline intravenously if the patient is unable to drink adequate fluids to prevent the severe dehydration that characterizes cholera.[184]

Charcoal Reactions in the Intestinal Tract

Charcoal reaches its maximal rate of adsorption extremely rapidly, within one minute. In thick or viscid fluids such as the intestinal or stomach juices, adsorption might be delayed somewhat, but can still be expected to be very rapid.[185]

In the past some have questioned the effects of the pH in the gastrointestinal tract on charcoal and its adsorbed materials, as to whether poisons might dissociate farther down and be absorbed into the blood. It has been found that charcoal forms a stable complex with toxic materials, and does not dissociate the toxins further down the gastrointestinal tract for later absorption into the blood stream.[186]

It has also been found that charcoal does not significantly adsorb nutrients. Two groups of rats were tested to determine if one group fed an identical diet with another group could be made to have deficiency disease by feeding charcoal. It was discovered that the two groups of rats were identical with or without charcoal.[187]

Charcoal added to the diet of sheep for 6 months did not cause a loss of nutrients, as compared with sheep not receiving charcoal. Blood tests showed no significant difference between the two groups of animals, and there were no visible signs of any nutritional deficiency. At

autopsy no differences either grossly or microscopically could be detected. A level of 5% of the total diet was given as charcoal. It did not affect the blood or urinary levels of calcium, copper, iron, magnesium, inorganic phosphorus, potassium, sodium, zinc, creatinine, uric acid, urea nitrogen, alkaline phosphatase, total protein or urine pH. It is of interest that although the animals inhaled some of the powdered charcoal, no ill effects could be demonstrated in the microscopic sections of the lungs and other structures of the chest.[188] Workers in charcoal manufacturing plants have been studied to determine the effect of breathing the dust of charcoal. It was found that the incidence of any respiratory symptoms was extremely low, suggesting that breathing the dust was quite innocuous.[189]

Ideally both vomiting and inactivation of the poison should be combined in the early treatment of acute poisonings. Syrup of Ipecac and apomorphine both bring up only about 30% of the poison in the stomach, meaning that they are inefficient in preventing poisoning by inducing vomiting, as 70% of the poison is retained in the stomach.

Lavage of the stomach is another method for treating poisoning, but the use of charcoal is far more effective and easy. It is non-toxic, and maintains its potency indefinitely in a closed container and can be conveniently and safely administered in the home. Activated charcoal is very well tolerated, even in amounts up to 100 grams (about 3/4 of a cupful of pulverized dry powder!) and there is no known contraindication to its use in acute poisonings. It is immediately effective and can be safely used by nonprofessionals. Charcoal is the most valuable single agent currently available for treating poisonings.[190] Babies and children accept slurries made of powdered activated charcoal. If enough charcoal is used there is almost no likelihood of dislodging the adsorbed material from the charcoal grains further down the digestive tract.

Charcoal adsorbs well at body temperature, but not so well at elevated temperatures. Heating in the oven causes substances that have been adsorbed to be released. Charcoal can be reused once or twice by washing, allowing to settle, pouring off the fluid and drying the charcoal in the oven at a high temperature (about 350°) but not high enough for the charcoal to ash.

Substances can be adsorbed from a water solution better than from an organic solvent. Salts such as sodium chloride and potassium nitrate are not readily adsorbed by activated charcoal. Iodine and mercuric chloride are well adsorbed. Simple acids and bases are easily adsorbed. Caustic materials are probably not readily adsorbed. In the swallowing of caustic agents such as lye, the offending agent may be poorly adsorbed unless large quantities of charcoal are used. While charcoal does no harm, it may not do much good, and more definitive treatment should be sought, such as drinking dilute vinegar solution. The same may be true of the alcohols, methanol, and ethanol, as there is experimental evidence in rats that charcoal is not effective in alcohol intoxication.[183]

On the skin, charcoal has been found to have no observable harmful effects. It will adsorb cancer-producing agents which, when free on the skin, are capable of producing skin cancer. It will effectively adsorb such known cancer-producing agents as methylcholanthrene and benzopyrene.[192]

Once a substance is adsorbed onto charcoal, washing with blood plasma or gastric juice will not cause the adsorbed material to desorb, the toxic material having been bound so firmly that it will not be removed by ordinary means.[193]

Substances Adsorbed by Charcoal[273]

Acetaminophen	Meprobamate
Aconitine	Mercuric chloride
Alcohol	Methylene blue
Amphetamine	Methyl salicylate
Antimony	Morphine
Antipyrine	Muscarin
Arsenic	Narcotics
Aspirin	Neguvon
Atropine	Nicotine
Barbital	Nortriptyline
Barbiturates	Opium
Cantharides	Parathion
Camphor	Penicillin
Chlordane	Pentobarbital
Chloroquine	Pesticides
Chlorpheniramine	Phenobarbital
Chlorpromazine	Phenolphthalein
Cocaine	Phenol
Colchicine	Phenylpropanolamine
Cyanide	Potassium cyanide
Delphinium	Potassium permaganate
2,4-Dichlorophenoxyacetic acid	Primaquine
Digitalis	Propantheline
Diphenylhydantoin	Propoxyphene
Diphenoxylates	Quinacrine
Elaterin	Quinidine
Ergotamine	Quinine
Ethchlorvynol	Radioactive substances
Gasoline	Salicylamide
Glutethimide	Salicylates
Hemlock	Secobarbital
Hexachlorophene	Selenium
Imipramine	Silver
Iodine	Stramonium
Ipecac	Strychnine
Isoniazid	Sulfonamides
Kerosene	Veratrine
Lead acetate	Some silver and
Malathion	antimony salts
Mefenamic acid	

The Charcoal Poultice

A charcoal poultice for a large area such as the abdomen or a knee joint, can be made as follows: 3 tablespoons flaxseed ground in a blender or seed mill, and mixed with 1-3 tablespoons of pulverized charcoal. Stir this mixture into one cup of water. Let it set for 10-20 minutes, or heat slightly to thicken.

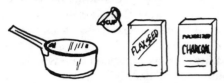

Put 3 tablespoons of charcoal and 3 tablespoons of flaxseed (congeals faster if it is first ground in a blender) in a pot with 1 cup of water. Bring to a boil while stirring. It becomes a gelatinous mixture.

Spread over a square of paper toweling of the proper size, using enough to make the paste 1/4 inch deep on the paper towel. Cover with another square of toweling. The edge of the poultice should not have paste spread on it for about 1/2 to 1 inch all around to minimize leakage. Place the poultice on the skin, cover with a piece of plastic that extends 1 inch over all edges and cover the entire plastic with an old towel to catch leaks that may develop. Use a binder or roller bandage to hold in place, pinning securely. Leave it on for 6-10 hours. Rub the area briskly with a cold washcloth after removing the compress.

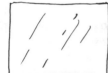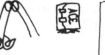

Kitchen plastic

Spread the thickened charcoal-flaxseed material over a piece of cotton cloth or double thickness paper towel. Cover with a single thickness cloth or paper towel. Lay the poultice over the affected area. Cover with plastic wrap, and hold in place by roller bandage such as strips of bed sheeting, an old towel, or an ace bandage. Pin securely with safety pins.

In order to make a poultice for a bee sting, spider bite or other venomous bite, simply dissolve a spoonful or more (determined by the size of the area to be treated and the seriousness of the affliction) of charcoal powder, or crush up several charcoal tablets in plain water, spread the paste over a folded piece of facial tissue or paper toweling, making the poultice fit the area to be treated, and molding the poultice over the area. The tissue or towel should be thoroughly moistened with the paste. The poultice can be molded around body parts, such as the ear when treating an earache, making the poultice fit the side of the jaw, the upper neck, as well as enclosing the ear lobe and skin behind the ear to the hairline.

Cover the poultice with a plastic piece cut from an ordinary bread bag, large enough to lap over all sides by at least one inch. Fix the poultice in place by a roller bandage, an ace bandage, or adhesive tape. A snug-fitting garment, such as a knitted cap, can be used over a charcoal compress to hold it on the eye or over the sinuses. A sweat shirt can help hold a charcoal compress snugly against the chest.

Charcoal Poultice with Hops or Smartweed

Make the poultice essentially the same as the plain charcoal poultice described above, but add to the paste fresh or dry commercial hops by simply crushing the leaves and adding them to the charcoal paste. Fresh leaves may be whirled in a blender a few seconds with a small amount of water before adding to the charcoal. To convert this poultice to a stupe, which may give a greater reaction, simply apply a moderately hot fomentation over the poultice and leave in place for about 20 minutes. Remove the fomentation, dry off any moisture and cover well with a sweater or snug fitting shirt for the night.

Charcoal and Flaxseed Poultice

Mix one tablespoon of charcoal powder in a cup with one tablespoon of flaxseed which has been ground in a blender. Add 1/3 cup of water and mix thoroughly. Bring to a boil, and use the thick material to spread on a linen piece or folded paper towel, as in the plain charcoal poultice.

Charcoal as an Antidote for Bites and Stings

Externally, venomous bites can be readily treated with charcoal. *Fire ants* leave a sterile abscess under the stings from the venom which kills a tiny area of tissue. An ordinary band-aid, wet slightly and rubbed with a charcoal tablet until it is entirely black, and applied as a mini-poultice combats ant stings. The same treatment is effective for mosquito bites, chigger bites, and poison ivy.

The perfect treatment for bee stings is a charcoal poultice. Many years ago we had a young co-worker who was stung on the finger by a yellow jacket. He spent one sleepless night due to pain, and was about to go into his second when he decided that he would apply a charcoal poultice. At that time none of us had used charcoal poultices for yellow jacket stings and didn't know what to expect. Within *five minutes* the pain was gone and he slept all night. Since that time whenever anyone is stung by a *bee, wasp,* or *yellow jacket,* we promptly apply a poultice which will prevent either swelling or pain.

A few years later a lady who had been told that she would probably die if she were ever stung again by a honey bee, received a *bee sting* on the thumb while walking near the home of a friend. Within two minutes she had begun to sweat all over, had developed a headache, and had severe pain in the thumb. A charcoal poultice was quickly applied and the general reaction entirely subsided within 5 minutes. Although she usually experienced massive swelling after bee stings, this time she had no trace of swelling. It is apparent that an anaphylactoid reaction was prevented in this lady by the charcoal poultice.

We have not had experience in treating *snakebites* with charcoal, but physicians who have successfully used it find it a good treatment. In isolated areas where antivenin is unavailable, and for snakebites for which there is no antivenin, we would immediately apply a very large charcoal poultice covering almost an entire extremity, centering over the bite, using large quantities of powdered charcoal wet with water, replacing the charcoal poultice about every 10 or 15 minutes.

The sooner the charcoal is applied, the more effective the treatment should be, as swelling in a snakebite begins within 10 minutes. We recommend that charcoal be carried in the pocket for first aid when individuals are hiking in snake-infested woods, so that the charcoal can be applied to any venomous bites promptly. Once swelling begins, the venom may not be able to transfer into the charcoal as easily. Ten charcoal tablets should be taken by mouth immediately. As long as the pain and swelling are being controlled by the poultices we would continue with this treatment alone. If pain and swelling should progress we would add ice packs to the extremity. Large quantities of charcoal should be taken periodically by mouth, as many poisons can be secreted into the gastrointestinal tract. Injections equivalent to 100 fatal doses of cobra venom had no venomous effect when activated charcoal was added to a solution of the venom and agitated before injection into experimental animals.

The treatment of choice for the *brown recluse spider* is charcoal. There is no other recognized treatment except wide surgical excision. There is no known antidote. The brown recluse spider produces a bite that gives little or no pain at first. In 24 hours a purplish red zone develops around the bite, and extensive tissue death occurs. It may produce a very deep and angry ulceration extending down to the bone, which lasts for weeks or months. We

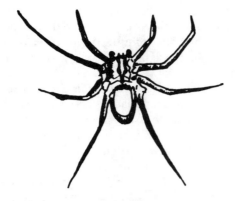

The Brown Recluse Spider. The spider is identified by the fiddle-shaped mark on the thorax.

have had three brown recluse spider bites successfully treated with charcoal, which produced no ulcerations and only the faintest purple discoloration after one week. The sooner treatment is begun the better. The spider is brown and has a fiddle-shaped mark on the back.

Specific Uses for Charcoal

1. Tylenol (Acetaminophen)

Acetaminophen poisoning can be treated with charcoal,[194] as can cobra venom, diphtherial toxin[195] and numerous ingested poisons.[196]

2. Aspirin

Activated charcoal used for aspirin poisoning is quite effective. In 1967, 17,995 cases of aspirin poisoning were reported, mostly involving children under five. Dozens of deaths result from such poisoning. Activated charcoal should be given promptly. In one study, when no activated charcoal was taken with a dose of aspirin, approximately 99.6% of the aspirin was absorbed from the gastrointestinal tract. The figure dropped to 58.9% in subjects given 10 grams (about 1 tablespoon) of activated charcoal immediately after taking aspirin. If the administration of activated charcoal was delayed one hour, the percentage absorbed rose sharply to 78.5%. When large amounts of aspirin are taken, activated charcoal is somewhat useful even up to 6 hours, but progressively less so.[197]

3. Bad Breath

Charcoal can be used for bad breath, cleansing both the mouth and the gastrointestinal tract. Even odor-producing substances that are secreted into the gastrointestinal tract high up will be adsorbed and their excretion through the lungs prevented. Odors produced in the mouth can be counteracted by proper cleansing of the teeth, tongue and gums by a soft bristle brush, and then holding a charcoal tablet in the mouth for 20-30 minutes.

4. Cancer

The anemia experienced in cancer can be treated with charcoal since this anemia is usually due to the toxins produced by cancer. The toxins are hemolytic and can be adsorbed onto the charcoal administered by mouth.[198] The pain produced by cancer can often be controlled by charcoal poultices. Pain in bone, abdomen, and elsewhere will often respond readily to charcoal poultices.

Charcoal poultices have been reported to completely check round cell sarcomas in dogs. Mouse cancer has not responded so well.[199]

5. Colostomy and Ileostomy Odor

As a fecal deodorant for patients who have ileostomies or colostomies, doctors have used activated charcoal routinely three times daily to reduce odors with good effect. Interestingly, only one-third of the patients continue this practice after five years, although initially they eagerly accept the treatment. It may be that they learn to handle the equipment better or become more skillful in avoiding certain foods that are more likely to cause odors. No apparent ill-effects from long term use have been described, even for these nutritionally marginal patients.[200]

6. Eye and Ear Conditions

The eyes are really another lobe of the brain. A treatment to the eyes can result also in a treatment to the brain, and it is well to remember that such afflictions of the brain as meningitis and encephalitis may respond somewhat to charcoal poultices and other treatments applied to the eyes.

Since inflamed tissue behind the eyes can become congested, if one level of temperature does not feel good to the eyes, change to another; if heat applied to the eyes does not feel good, change to cold, or the other way around. Often that which feels most agreeable will be the most effective treatment.

Cellulitis of the face, eyelids and ears can be effectively treated with a poultice of charcoal. Otitis media or otitis externa can be treated by a charcoal poultice

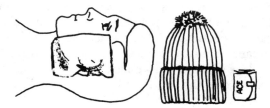

Charcoal poultice for earache. Mold the charcoal poultice over the ear and allow it to extend downward onto the neck, forward over the jaw, and upward to the hairline. Hold the poultice in place with an ace bandage and a knit cap pulled down well over the face and ears. Relief of earache often begins in 4-5 minutes.

molded over the exterior of the ear.[201] A heat lamp used over the poultice to keep it warm can increase its effectiveness. Keep moistening the poultice under the drying lamp.

7. Intestinal Gas, Diarrhea, Indigestion

Flatulence and abdominal distention can be readily treated with charcoal to good advantage. Use 4 capsules or 8 tablets as often as 3 or 4 times a day. Nervous diarrhea with irritable or *spastic colon* is greatly helped by taking charcoal. For bed patients who produce malodorous stools, charcoal can be a great assistance.[202] For indigestion, use powdered charcoal stirred into a little olive oil for cleansing and healing.

For *indigestion, peptic ulcers,* or other forms of gastrointestinal distress, the fluid resulting after charcoal has been stirred into water and allowed to settle may be

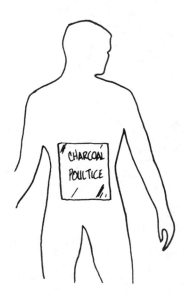

For abdominal pain lay a poultice of charcoal over the abdomen. In half an hour severe pain is often entirely relieved.

quite helpful. Stir about 1 tablespoon of charcoal into a large glass of water and allow the black part to settle to the bottom. The slurry water on top may be drunk with good results. Visible particles in suspension may be observed by shining a light obliquely through the water. Patients who are already taking a moderate amount of charcoal may benefit from taking their drinking water in this form. Patients with *ulcerative colitis* fall in this category, as well as some children who refuse to drink the black liquid. Persons with peptic ulcers and other very sensitive persons who get irritation from taking the whole charcoal may receive benefit from drinking slurry water.

8. Infections

Activated charcoal can adsorb bacteria, viruses, bacterial toxins, and hormones. Charcoal has been reported to disinfect wounds, and to act as a deodorizer in various bodily ills.[203] Charcoal can be used for wound dressings.[204]

On the body surface, charcoal will adsorb wound secretions, bacteria, carcinogens, toxins, products of allergies, and will reduce swelling by taking up excess tissue fluid and products of inflammation. Charcoal works better in an acid than in an alkaline medium. Charcoal has been used internally in Asiatic cholera, dysentery, diarrhea, and dyspepsia.[205]

Foot and mouth disease virus in a 1% suspension can be entirely adsorbed on charcoal if used in the amount of 10 grams of charcoal per 100 milliliters of fluid. The virus is not destroyed, but its activity is much reduced. Wood and coconut charcoal are less effective than bone charcoal for adsorbing foot and mouth disease virus. Sheep-pox virus is adsorbed on bone charcoal effectively.[206]

Suspensions of colloidal charcoal have been used intravenously in 100 cases of septicemia, metritis, mastitis, lymphangitis, and pyogenic wounds. After the infusion of charcoal there was seen an increase in the number of neutrophils. Elevated body temperatures returned to normal within one hour. The charcoal reportedly is filtered out in spleen, lymph nodes, liver, and other reticuloendothelial areas. Since patients receiving intravenous charcoal have sometimes experienced shortness of breath, it seems proper to say that capillaries in the lungs were plugged by the charcoal, at least temporarily. These patients were treated with intravenous injections of 0.001 grams per kilogram of body weight.[207] While we believe the intravenous use is contraindicated because of its obvious physiologic implications, it is interesting that it was at one time used successfully in this way to treat infections.

Since charcoal increases the intestinal transit time in some individuals, it is properly used in diarrhea. Bauer reported in 1928 that the administration of charcoal to experimental animals doubles transit time.[208]

9. Inflammation

We have had cases of cellulitis that have been painful, feverish and throbbing. It is no exaggeration to say that within 5 minutes after putting on a charcoal poultice the patient feels relaxed and in complete comfort. It is a miraculous thing to witness this reaction.

E. G. White once said, "One of the most beneficial remedies is pulverized charcoal in a bag, and used in fomentations. This is a most successful remedy; if wet smartweed is boiled, it is better still. I have ordered this in cases where the sick were suffering great pain before the close of life. When I suggested charcoal, and the patient has slept, the turning point came, and recovery was the result. To students, when injured with bruised hands, and suffering with inflammation, I have prescribed this simple remedy with perfect success. The poison of the inflammation is overcome, the pain removed and the healing went on rapidly. The more severe inflammation of the eyes will be relieved by a poultice of charcoal, put in a bag, and dipped in hot or cold water as will best suit the case. This works like a charm. I expect you to laugh at this, but if I could give this remedy some outlandish name, that no one knew but myself, it would have greater influence."[209]

10.   An Insecticide

Activated charcoal and clay samples have shown insecticidal activity. Activated charcoal has high levels of insecticidal activity even at 95% relative humidity, and 30°C. The insecticidal effectiveness increases with the fineness of the particles and the hardness number.[210]

11.   Jaundice

The need for exchange transfusion in babies with erythroblastosis fetalis has been cut by more than 90% with the use of charcoal. All jaundiced newborn babies with a serum bilirubin over 10 milligrams may be given 0.5 grams (about 1/2 teaspoon) of charcoal in sufficient water to pass through a nipple every 2-3 hours. Since serum bilirubin usually reaches 20 milligrams percent before an exchange transfusion takes place, the charcoal regimen affords an earlier therapy, and will often stabilize the bilirubin at much less than 20 milligrams.[211]

Neonatal jaundice, caused by an excess of bilirubin in the blood, is relatively frequent in infants, particularly those that are premature or those that are breastfed. Normally, a large quantity of blood is broken down in the first few days of life, putting quite a load of work on the liver. At this time the liver is still immature and cannot process a great load of broken down blood cells. Breastfeeding enhances jaundice of the newborn, since a hormone in milk retards the processing of bilirubin by the liver. We believe that a small elevation of the serum bilirubin is actually stimulatory to the developing brain, but excessive levels—over 25—may be injurious, although recent studies seem to implicate low oxygen rather than high bilirubin as the cause of kernicterus. Charcoal adsorbs bilirubin well from the duodenal fluid. One gram per day causes only part of the bilirubin to be bound, but 4.5 grams (2-3 teaspoons) per day of charcoal prevents all but a small amount of bilirubin from being absorbed from the duodenum. If charcoal feeding is started at 12 hours of age it is less effective than when the charcoal is begun at 4 hours of age, as the enterohepatic circulation of bilirubin may play a critical role in determining the size of the bilirubin pool during the first few hours of life.

The very first case of neonatal jaundice on which we used charcoal was a breastfed baby who developed jaundice on the fourth day of life. The baby was sent to the

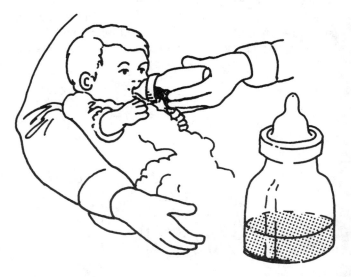

For erythroblastosis (jaundice in the newborn), put a tablespoon (about 4-8 grams) of pulverized charcoal in a nursing bottle with sufficient water to make a slurry barely capable of passing through the nipple. Shake well to blend. Start giving the charcoal water in suspected cases before the baby is 4 hours old. When combined with daily exposure to sunlight, bilirubin levels remain sufficiently low that most exchange transfusions can be avoided.

laboratory with his father, and the first total bilirubin level was 12 mg % on the 5th day, 14.5 mg. % twelve hours later, and 16 mg % 6 hours after that. A consultant agreed with our suspicion of an ABO incompatibility. At this point we began 6 hourly bilirubin determinations and appropriate associated laboratory tests. When the bilirubin rose to 18 mg % the consultant prepared for an exchange transfusion. That same hour the mother began administering as much charcoal as she could get the baby to accept and sat in the sunlight with the baby undressed in her lap, giving over an hour of exposure to both front and back (babies can tolerate more sunlight before getting a sunburn than can adults). At the next 6 hour bilirubin check the level was down to 16.5 mg % and we knew we had avoided the hazardous exchange transfusion. Continuing with this treatment the bilirubin began to clear and was down to 4 mg % by the 10th day.

12.   Kerosene, Gasoline, Lighter Fluid Ingestion

Charcoal can adsorb some gasoline, kerosene, lighter fluids, and cleaning fluids that children may accidently ingest, which may cause an involvement of the lungs and central nervous system. Since charcoal is not as efficient in adsorbing these substances, a much larger quantity of charcoal in relation to the offending fluid should be swallowed than for other poisons.

13.   Liver Failure

Patients with hepatic failure can be treated even in the home, but especially by hemoperfusion through columns of charcoal which extract most amino acids, drugs, and toxins from plasma. Individuals who have acute liver failure should be given large quantities of charcoal by mouth in an attempt to prevent toxins from building up in the blood.[213]

14.   Metabolic Problems

Orally administered activated charcoal given for 4-8 weeks to six adults suffering from renal insufficiency showed that their serum triglycerides fell an average of 36% and serum cholesterol by an average of 67%. Urea, uric acid, and creatine were not significantly affected. It is felt that the direct binding of lipids and bile acids in the intestine by charcoal produces these results. Itching in patients on longterm dialysis can be relieved by charcoal by mouth.[171]

15.   Mushroom Poisoning

Mushroom poisoning can be effectively treated with charcoal, even 24 hours after eating *Amanita phalloides*.[215] Unconscious patients can be given activated charcoal by gastric tube.[216]

16.   Pain

For abdominal pain use pulverized charcoal on the abdomen as a poultice, laying it over the entire abdomen and sides. Often great pain can be relieved in a short while by the use of charcoal poultices on the abdomen.

The pain of sore throat, earache, sprains, arthritis, pleurisy, and all other pains should be given a trial of a charcoal poultice. The pain that may have gone unabated for hours is often relieved in ten minutes.

17.   Theophyllin

Theophyllin, which is often given for respiratory tract problems in children, has a very narrow therapeutic index before toxic range is reached. Frequent acute overdoses can be expected, especially among children, since there is increased usage of this drug. Physicians and parents who prescribe and use drugs that can be dangerous to children should always have on hand activated charcoal ready for immediate administration.

18.   Women's Diseases

In 1930 Nahmacher reported on his experience with charcoal. He stated that he had treated spontaneous abortions by watchful management, unless hemorrhage required surgical interference. Only in criminal abortions, produced by external interference, did he see fever. In numerous abortion cases having admission temperatures up to 100.4, he was able to prove that in almost all cases the temperature fell to normal in 24 hours at most, and convalescence was entirely free of fever when granulated charcoal was introduced into the uterus through the cervix by means of one or two charcoal pencils. He assumed that bacteria in the uterine cavity had been adsorbed into the charcoal. He reported convalescence free from fever, in contradistinction to cases not treated with charcoal, in which a low grade fever extended over several days, indicating endometritis. He reports almost immediate cessation of a malodorous discharge in infected abortions treated with charcoal.

He reported that fever after the birth of a baby was very favorably influenced by intrauterine charcoal therapy. As soon as a foul smelling discharge and low grade fever set in, the patients were treated five to six days with certain medicines, an ice bag, raising the head of the bed 25 cm. (about 8 inches) to aid escape of the discharge, and if no improvement occurred, charcoal was introduced into the uterus on the seventh day under the strictest aseptic precautions. In all cases a reduction in temperature occurred the day following and was normal by the second day. The odor disappeared at once. In over 90% of cases it was unnecessary to insert charcoal pencils more than once.

The technique for insertion is as follows:

1. Cleanse the vaginal opening and the vagina. Insert a vaginal speculum.
2. Hook the anterior lip of the uterine cervix and cleanse the cervix of mucus and pus.
3. Grasp the charcoal pencil with a dressing forceps, dip two or three times in sterile water, and carefully insert it through the cervical canal to beyond the internal os. There is no need to dilate the os. Two or three pencils may be introduced if the uterine cavity is large enough, one toward the right, the second toward the left, and the third in the midline. A gauze is left against the os.[217]

"Always study and teach the use of the simplest remedies, and the special blessing of the Lord may be expected to follow the use of these means which are within the reach of the common people."[218]

The gastrointestinal tract is one of the most important systems for the removal of toxins, the lungs, skin, and urinary systems being the other routes of excretion of toxins. As materials are secreted from the blood into the gastrointestinal tract, the toxins may be either digested, or reabsorbed into the blood stream. If charcoal is present in the gastrointestinal tract, the toxic substances may adsorb into the charcoal. Since toxins may be actively secreted into the gastrointestinal tract from the blood stream, charcoal makes a very efficient cleanser of the blood when taken orally. Undigested vegetable fiber from fruits, vegetables and whole grains also act as material to adsorb toxins and prevent their absorption into the blood stream. It is believed that many cancer-producing chemicals leave the body in this manner.

Kaolin, a white clay, is another material that adsorbs substances from the gastrointestinal tract, and has been used in various preparations for gastrointestinal disorders (Kaopectate is an example.) Ordinary clay from the hillside can be used either externally or internally in the same manner as charcoal. It has been in use for centuries in Europe and Central America, but has had only limited use in the United States, mainly for bee stings and other venomous bites. Clay poutices have been used for boils, corns, callouses, hemorrhoids, ringworm, pinkeye, acne, gangrene, and skin sores and ulcers.

Internally clay has been used for constipation, and conversely for diarrhea. Just mix some clay with water and drink it, or make a paste—1-4 tablespoons of clay with enough water to moisten. Clay has been used as an antidote for poisons and for anemia.

To obtain the clay, go to an uninhabited area or in your backyard, dig down under the topsoil with a hoe or shovel, and take up the underlying clay. Be certain no chemicals have been dumped in the area, and that pesticides and herbicides have not been used. Sterilize the clay and dry it out by baking in an oven at 350° for 15-30 minutes until completely dry. Pound with a hammer if necessary to make the clay fine. May be stored for years without losing potency.[219]

CHAPTER SIXTEEN

Garlic And Its Relatives Used As Medicinal Herbs

Cultivation of Garlic, Its Commerce and Chemistry

Garlic grows like onion and may be easily cultivated in the garden. Both onion and garlic will survive most winter weather. The leaves, as well as the roots, may be eaten either raw or cooked, in the same way that onion is used. It has been suggested that companion planting of garlic between rows of vegetables or flowers would prevent insect infestation. This may be true in some areas, but we have not been able to detect this property of garlic in either orchard or garden. Twelve to fifteen plants around one tree failed to protect the tree from the usual insects.

Active Principles in Garlic

Garlic, Allium sativum L., contains a number of sulfides, the most active principle apparently being the allylthiosulfinicallyl ester, allicin.[213]

The chemical attributes of garlic that could influence its use as a therapeutic agent include a number of sulfur-containing compounds; a number of minerals: manganese, copper, iron, zinc, calcium, aluminum and selenium; and the specific factor, allicin. Allicin is the strongly odorous substance of garlic, being converted to alliin by alliinase. The essential oil of garlic can produce approximately 60% of its weight in allicin after exposure to the enzyme. Heat destroys the enzyme alliinase, accounting for the fact that cooked garlic does not produce the strong odor of raw garlic. Since certain forms of allicin-like compounds are present only in the raw state, some therapeutic properties are dependent on the use of raw garlic. Aliin is stable in storage for long periods in both the aqueous extract and in the dehydrated garlic powder. Allicin in aqueous extract is not stable during storage and loses its antibacterial activity.[221] [222]

Garlic is especially high in selenium, possibly the best vegetable source of this trace element. Selenium stimulates the immune response, and acts in the same antioxidant way as vitamin E. Thus the antioxidant quality of garlic should make it an excellent anti-aging factor, by interfering with the formation of "free radicals," the particles formed by the action of atmospheric radiation and ozone on polyunsaturated oils in the cells. Its immune stimulating abilities could be useful in allergies and infections.[223]

Garlic can be obtained in pill form, both the dried whole garlic and the oil of garlic. Garlic pills are usually taken in dosage of two or three about three times a day. When using the raw cloves of garlic, one to three small cloves in one meal are sufficient, and more may be undesirable. In most cases one clove per meal or even one clove per day may be all that is needed. Over-using any food or nutrient can result in unpleasant symptoms. I do not know of any unpleasant symptoms that arise from the use of garlic, but common sense would indicate that its overuse would be undesirable.

Except in tropical areas, Aloe vera should be grown in pots as house plants, or in the greenhouse, as they do not tolerate frost. Every home should have an aloe plant growing in the kitchen. The commercial forms of Aloe vera are as liquid, gel, creams, shampoo, capsules, etc.

Garlic has been shown to have a significant protective action against hyperlipemia and blood coagulation. Onion also helps prevent high blood lipids.[224]

The cholesterol and blood lipid-lowering effect of garlic is attributed to the presence of diallyldisulphide.[265] [266] Other therapeutic effects that have been attributed to garlic are anti-hemolytic and anti-arthritic factors, sugar regulation, anti-oxidant, anticoagulant, antibacterial, antifungal and antiviral properties. Such diseases as intestinal and skin parasites, fungus skin infections, hoof and mouth disease, colds and influenza (both to prevent and to treat), constipation, asthma (and other respiratory disorders such as emphysema and whooping cough) high blood pressure, tuberculosis, diabetes, and insomnia have all been successfully treated with garlic. Anemia has been studied using garlic as a treatment. In one study, after eight weeks of treatment with garlic extract or cooked garlic (best not raw in anemia), there was shown a very nice improvement in the hemoglobin. Feeding fresh raw onion juice to rats and dogs caused a decrease in the number of red blood cells and an increase in the number of white blood cells.[225]

Uses Ascribed to Garlic

Acne
Allergies
Anemia
Angina
Antispasmotic-colic of both infants and adults. Use a small dose for babies—1/4 teaspoon of minced, fresh or dry granules in 3 ounces of water.
Arteriosclerosis
Arthritis
Athlete's foot
Blood clots inside veins
Cancer
Childbirth problems
Colds
Colitis
Concentration, poor
Coughs
Cryptococcus infections—an old Chinese remedy used in "enormous quantities" by mouth
Cystitis—excreted in the urine (Combats infection: Use 3 large cloves 3 times daily for five days)
Diabetes—to reduce the blood sugar, and to combat the complications of diabetes
Digestive disorders
Diuretic
Dizziness
Dysentery
Eczema
Expectorant (asthma, whooping cough, bronchitis)
Fats high in the blood
Headache
Heart disease
Heavy metal poisoning
Hemorrhoids[267]
High blood pressure—dilates blood vessels and reduces high blood pressure
Hypoglycemia[268]
Influenza and colds, both prevention and treatment
Insect repellent
Intestinal gas
Intestinal parasites in dogs and man
Lupus erythematosus
Plague, cholera, typhus—Use 1/2 teaspoon garlic oil blended in 1 pint water; also as nosedrops or gargle solution for irrigations
Plantar warts—oil rubbed in daily, or used as a fresh garlic—mini-poultice

Polio
Poultices for dermatitis, boils, abscesses, sores
Pyorrhea
Respiratory disorders
Sciatica
Sore throat as a lozenge—1 slice of garlic on each side of the mouth between cheek and teeth. Colds and sore throat treated with garlic often disappear in a few hours.
Tuberculosis

A cancer-inhibiting factor has been reported in garlic. Generally a substance that contains a grouping of atoms in the following arrangement, -SO-S-S, is associated with the inhibition of cell growth, whereas cell division and mitosis are promoted by sulfhydryl (-SH) groupings. Any agent that attaches or oxidizes sulfhydryl compounds inhibits cell division. Allicin has been found to inhibit sulfhydryl enzymes. Sulfhydryl-deficient diets may inhibit tumor growth in some animals. Contrariwise, the addition of the amino acid cysteine or glutathione which contain the -SH grouping, may have the opposite effect. It has been reported that pure alliin has growth inhibiting characteristics on various tumors. Synthetic alliin, however, was found ineffective. Further, it has been noted in human luekemia that the metabolism of sulfhydryl compounds is abnormal. These facts led in 1960 to a study to evaluate the effect of alliin and allicin upon mouse tumors. If the tumors were incubated in a test tube with allicin prior to transplanting there was complete inhibition of tumor growth. The results of the rest of this study were disappointing, however, in that single or multiple treatments to the mouse itself with either allicin or alliin did not produce any consistent and significant tumor inhibition, even when large doses of 30 mg. per kg. were given. Garlic extract was similar in producing no inhibition of tumor growth when the animal itself received the garlic.[226]

Mice exposed to cancer cells that had been treated with garlic did not die of cancer, but those mice exposed to cancer cells which were untreated died within a month. [227] Scordinin and germanium are both considered to be anti-cancer substances and both occur in garlic.

Germanium is an oxygen carrier reportedly producing an invigorating effect on healthy and ill alike. Germanium produces no known side-effects, no genetic changes, but apparently acts as an anti-cancer agent. Some studies in Japan on the influence of germanium on cancer in rats show some promise.[228]

Intestinal Parasites

Feeding garlic to humans or dogs infested with hookworms significantly reduces the number of larvae grown

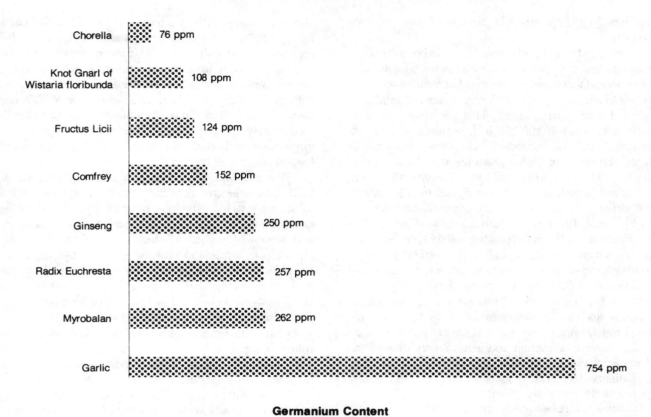

**Germanium Content
Of Various Herbs**

from fecal material in cultures. During a period that both dogs and man were taking small doses of garlic, the number of eggs found in the stool was not significantly affected on three teaspoons of minced garlic daily. Perhaps the dosage needs to be 6 teaspoons or more of raw minced garlic daily.[229]

Antivirus Properties

In the 1918 flu epidemic, about twenty people in one area experimented with taking garlic daily in the meals. None of the twenty had the flu.

Antifungus Properties

Frozen cloves of garlic were blended thoroughly with water, incubated at 37° for one hour, and used against several fungi which cause skin lesions in humans. The garlic water was able to inhibit the growth of Microsporum gypseum, Trichophyton verrucosum, Trichophyton violaceum, Trichophyton rubrum, Trichophyton schoenleini, Trichophyton mentagrophytes, and Epidermophyton floccosum. Guinea pigs and rabbits infected with these fungi produced ex-

cellent healing in 14-17 days with twice daily applications of the garlic water for only one week. It can be said that garlic showed a fungicidal effect in these experiments.[230]

Antimicrobial Factors

Inhibition of bacterial growth by garlic, onion, and aloe vera has been suggested by some experiments. The antibacterial principle of garlic can be easily prepared for use from the cloves, and has been demonstrated to be effective against gram positive, gram negative, acid fast and fungal organisms.[231] Studies to demonstrate the bacterial growth-inhibiting properties of onion juice using the yellow globe and white onions showed inhibition of bacterial growth when the filtered juice was incorporated in a fluid medium. It was effective in preventing the growth of Bacillus subtilis. Heating weakened the potency of the juice, although cold storage for four months had no effect.[232]

Garlic has been used to treat cryptococcal meningitis. Garlic did not result in quite as high a percentage of recoveries as with amphotericin B, but the side effects of amphotericin B are severe, and often disabling. With garlic nearly a 70% effective treatment rate was obtained.[233]

A crude extract of garlic was found to be quite effective against gram negative as well as gram positive bacteria in bacterial culture. Even those bacteria which were resistant to commonly used antibiotics showed inhibition of growth with garlic extract. This property was completely inactivated at 100° C. in five minutes. Oral administration of the extract to chickens considerably reduced the count of viable gram negative bacteria normally present in the intestinal tract. The growth of proteus but not pseudomonas was inhibited in culture.[234]

A distinct beneficial action is exerted on intestinal flora by garlic, favoring an increase in aciduric growth and retardation of the gram positive proteolytic types. Indicanuria when present, an index of intestinal putrefaction, disappeared when 22 human subjects were treated with desiccated garlic in therapeutic doses.[235]

Garlic has been used in India against leprosy. Garlic by mouth and in an ointment used on four patients showed much improvement in lesions or complete clearing. The nerve dysfunction and general condition of the patients were much improved after 24 weeks of therapy. The patients felt well and showed no unfavorable response to the garlic treatment.[236]

Biostymin, a substance found in aloe vera, acts as a biologic stimulator in allergic and infectious diseases. A beneficial effect in various diseases is believed by investigators to be due to a stimulatory reaction in the adrenals, spleen, and reticuloendothelial tissues. The increased production of glycoproteid immune bodies by the reticulum cells, and the increased hormonal activity of the adrenal cortex and the adrenal medulla appear to be the means of benefit in such diseases as asthma.[237]

Aloe vera contains an active principle for promoting healing, thought by some to be a mucopolysaccharide. Aloe vera has been shown to be helpful in the treatment of chronic leg ulcers; baldness, both spot baldness and falling hair; and in acne.

Allicin is a potent antibacterial agent.[206] Garlic juice inhibited the growth of Staphylococcus aureus, Escherichia coli, and Candida albicans, the latter being most sensitive and S. aureus showing the next greatest sensitivity.[238] A sulfur-containing antibiotic in garlic is known to be effective against a wide variety of bacteria. The antimicrobial action of garlic is ascribed by investigators to the presence of numerous sulfides, inhibiting the cellular activity of Streptococcus pyogenes, Salmonella typhosa, and Bacterium dysenteriae.[240]

Some investigators pinpoint an aldehyde as apparently the active principle in garlic which accounts for its antibacterial action. At room temperature the material is stable for months, at 37° C. for several hours, and shows no loss in activity after heating at 55° C. for half an hour or 75° C. for 15 minutes. Heating at 75° C. for half an hour caused a slight loss, and more marked loss after one hour. Boiling for a few seconds or heating at 100° C. for one minute causes a marked loss in potency, and the activity is totally destroyed after exposure to this temperature for half an hour. Any alkali will inactivate the medicinal principle. These properties correspond to a large extent to those of allicin. The active principle is both bacteriostatic and bacteriocidal.

It was found that in high dilutions garlic juice actually enhances growth of bacteria. A one to two hundred dilution seems to be the most potent stimulator. The question is raised whether high dilutions might also raise the resistance of the host to infection. Tests on rabbits and guinea pigs artificially infected with various organisms failed to show an advantage for those animals treated with garlic, except that the treated animals had a delay in death in a few instances. There could be a narrow margin between the therapeutic and the toxic doses.[241]

Garlic can be used as a bacteriostatic agent, a preparation being used as an antiseptic.[242]

Garlic juice and garlic poultices could be used in the treatment of active chronic skin ulcers.[243]

While using a method for the assay of penicillin, certain plant extracts were also tested for antibacterial activity. It was discovered that ground garlic cloves possessed high antibacterial activity. It is equally effective against gram positive and gram negative organisms.[244]

Soothes the Digestive Tracts

Garlic has been suggested as a laxative, for painful flatulence, and for abdominal complaints following the use of alcohol. A garlic-charcoal preparation administered for one month definitely reduced symptoms, and relieved signs of intestinal and gastric flatulence, as well as abdominal distention.[245]

Garlic concentrate loses its efficiency when administered continuously. It should be administered for three days, skipping the fourth. Some say that when used with parsley powder, the characteristic odor of garlic is neutralized. Others say this is not true. The tablets should be swallowed, and not chewed, however.

Female Disorders and Endocrine Disturbances Treated with Garlic

Such gynecologic disorders as painful menstruation and menopausal problems have been favorably treated with garlic.[246] Water extracts of garlic possess a biologically active thyroid -like material.[247]

Asthma Treated with Garlic

An effective treatment for acute asthma consists of the preparation of two cups of hot water at about 105° F. into which two garlic cloves have been thoroughly blended. The addition of a small amount of salt may make the dose more palatable. The first cupful should be drunk rapidly. In some individuals the hot garlic water may cause vomiting. In asthma, this is a good treatment, as vomiting loosens bronchial plugs and encourages watery secretions and coughing. Many times the vomiting alone is accompanied by marked relief. Nevertheless, the second cup of the garlic mixture is administered promptly after vomiting, during the "refractory phase," when vomiting usually will not occur. In this way the second cup can generally be retained. The active principle in garlic is excreted in the lungs, adding the beneficial effects of the aromatic garlic principles in loosening of secretions. The odor of garlic can be detected on the breath within 20 to 30 minutes. Use this treatment with the treatments in the hydrotherapy section suggested for asthma.

Heart, Arteries and Blood Pressure

Dr. Hans Reuter of Cologne and other researchers in Bonn, West Germany suggest the use of garlic in preventing heart attacks.[248] It is known that garlic oil significantly inhibits the production of high blood cholesterol in rabbits fed a diet designed to produce increased tissue and blood cholesterol. The arteriosclerosis was reduced to about one-fourth the amount in the control group. [249] The presence of atheromatous changes in the aorta were minimized by the administration of garlic oil. The material used was the oil fraction extracted from raw garlic. While the garlic did not completely prevent the increase in tissue and blood cholesterol, it did significantly reduce the effect.[250] The results of one feeding experiment "suggest that garlic reduces lipid synthesis and influences glycogen metabolism in the liver of rats."[251]

The mustard oil of garlic is said to dilate arteries and veins. Such an effect would have a salutary result on high blood pressure by reducing the peripheral resistance to blood flow.

Headaches and dizziness associated with high blood pressure clear when garlic is administered.[252] Garlic has both a direct and indirect hypotensive action. The indirect effect is by checking intestinal putrefaction. It may be this blood vessel dilating effect that gives the reported diuresis with onion. A congestive heart failure patient ate an onion daily and had a good diuresis.[253]

Garlic as an Anticoagulant

Onion and garlic extracts contain substances which inhibit platelet aggregation.[254] This aggregation is essential to the formation of an effective clot. This means that onion and garlic may help prevent formation of blood clots in the brain, heart, and extremities. It can be recommended that persons who are susceptible to easy clotting within their arteries eat these commonly used dietary articles as a means of preventing clots. Platelets of the blood are produced in the bone marrow as are blood cells. Platelets have to do with clotting of the blood. Prior to the formation of a blood clot, the platelets stick together in clusters to aid in the development of the clot.

There are several features of life style that tend to promote excessively easy clotting of the blood: overeating, the use of a large quantity of dietary fat, lack of exercise, lying down immediately after a meal, etc. Onion and garlic have been shown to reduce the stickiness of platelets and to retard abnormally brisk clotting action. This feature of onions would be particularly desirable in persons who tend to form clots inside their veins. Those who have heart or artery disease are likely to produce intravascular clots. These include diabetics, those with high levels of cholesterol or triglycerides, high blood pressure, and rhythm disturbances of the heart. The factor which reduces platelet stickiness is stable even after heating, indicating that cooked onion and garlic would also be effective in keeping down blood clots.[255]

Six healthy adults showed that the clumping together of platelets caused by certain substances (ADP, epinephrine and collagen) was inhibited by both injections of the essential oil of garlic, as well as the oral administration of garlic. It would seem proper to expect that garlic as well as onion would have properties to inhibit clot formation in the body.[256]

It has been reported that eating cooked onions can stop the bleeding and discomfort of hemorrhoids. One person reported that on days cooked onions were eaten no bleeding occurred. If onions were not eaten daily bleeding from the hemorrhoids was the rule.[257]

It is recognized that dietary fats increase the likelihood of intravascular clotting by reducing fibrinolytic activity of the blood. Several investigators have shown that this reduction in fibrinolytic activity from a high fat diet can be prevented by eating onions steamed or boiled. In fact, onions actually increase the fibrinolytic activity of the blood, making blood clots within the veins less likely. Persons in danger of excessive clotting should eat onions for their fibrinolytic action.[258] [259]

An occasional voice against garlic is heard. One writer incorrectly states that foods should not be used to supply the need for medicine. Many foods have properties that can be readily used to correct a situation that might otherwise require a medicine—the cabbage family for hyperthyroidism, and the foods high in plant steroids for menopausal symptoms. Since garlic contains certain substances having well-defined properties, the pharmacologic effect of these substances may not be desirable on a regular and long term basis. Nevertheless, for a few days or weeks, or intermittently on an indefinite basis would not seem undesirable. Mustard oil in garlic is an indigestible drug and pervades tissues and cells, requiring the body to eliminate it through the kidneys and lungs. It is suggested that its long-term use might injure these organs, but no studies are known to substantiate this idea.

The common onion has been reported to have a hypoglycemic effect.[270] Tests to clarify this matter were done on rabbits. Extracts of dried onions were given to normal male rabbits having a fasting 18 hour blood sugar level of 100 mg% to 120mg%. The potency of these extracts was determined. There was a mean reduction in the blood sugar of from 15.5% to 19.2% after giving 0.5 grams of a petroleum extract or ethyl ether extract. The study confirmed that Allium cepa, the common onion, does have hypoglycemic properties. In a feeding study involving rats, a "garlic diet significantly reduced serum glucose but increased serum insulin and liver glycogen . . . The hypoglycemic effect of garlic seems associated with the increase of insulin level."[260]

Garlic has been found to kill mosquito larvae.[261] The crushed raw garlic can be stirred into a quart of water and sprinkled over open pools containing larvae.

Use of Aloe Vera

The uses of Aloe vera are almost identical to those of garlic and onion, but perhaps a simple listing will emphasize the importance of Aloe vera in home remedies. Aloe vera liquid has been successfully used on burns, infected wounds, poison ivy, insect stings, shingles, fever blisters, diaper rash, x-ray burns, abscesses, mouth ulcers, sore throat, pyorrhea, peptic ulcers, colitis, constipation, diverticulitis, arthritis, liver diseases, skin problems (fungus diseases, warts, rashes, psoriasis, acne, dry skin, callouses, sunburn, any dermatitis) and itching.

The thick gel from the leaves can be used as a shampoo by rubbing it into the scalp and hair the night before shampooing. The treatment is said to be good for dandruff and other scalp conditions. Do not use soap as the aloe foams nicely, and soap and soap shampoos are not good for dandruff. No conditioner is needed as the hair is left soft, shiny, and manageable after the aloe application.

GLOSSARY

ABO incompatibility—Blood type incompatibility similar to Rh incompatibility.

Acclimatization—Becoming accustomed to a climate.

Acetaminophen—Tylenol.

Acidosis—The condition of being acid.

Adaptive mechanisms—Adjustments made to stress.

Agglutinins—Substances that cause cells to stick together.

Aldosterone—A hormone produced in the adrenals which elevates blood pressure.

Alkalinity—Pertaining to the state of being alkaline.

Alkaloids—A group of toxic chemicals of which caffeine is a member.

Allergens—Substances that stimulate an allergy.

Allopathy—The branch of healing arts using drugs and surgery as the major treatment modality. The word means inducing an opposite kind of reaction than that produced by the body.

Anastomosis—A communication, usually between arteries and veins.

Anodyne—A pain reliever.

Antigens—Substances foreign to the body which stimulate an antibody response.

Antivenin—Antibodies made artificially which neutralize poisons, such as snake venom.

Aorta—The largest artery in the body, arising from the heart.

Arterioles—Very small arteries.

Asiatic cholera—A serious disease characterized by diarrhea and fever.

Autonomic nervous system—The "automatic nervous system," made up of the sympathetic and parasympathetic nervous systems.

Bacteriocidal agent—A substance which kills bacteria.

Bacteriostatic agent—An agent which stops the growth of bacteria.

Candida albicans—A yeast producing various infections in the body such as thrush.

Capillaries—Very small blood vessels which connect to the smallest arteries on one side and the smallest veins on the other.

Capillary permeability—The ability of substances to pass through the wall of a capillary.

Carbuncles—An abscess with many heads.

Carcinogens—Cancer producing agents.

Cardiotonic—A substance increasing the tone of the heart.

Carditis—An inflammation of the heart.

Carotid arteries—The large arteries of the neck carrying blood to the face and head.

Catabolic action—Forces in the body that break down.

Catatonia—A serious form of mental illness characterized by a pronounced slowing of movements.

Cholera—(see Asiatic cholera)

Chondrosarcoma—A malignant tumor of cartilage.

Chorea—A disorder characterized by involuntary movements.

Circadian Rhythm—The biologic time clock.

Conjunctiva—The thin membrane that lines the eyelids and covers the outer portion of the eye.

Connective tissue—Tissue which supports and connects other body tissues.

Cryptococcus—A fungus causing systemic disease.

Dander—Animal dandruff or other material shed from skin.

Dermis—The deep layer of skin.

Dermatitis—An inflammation of the skin.

Dermatomyositis—A collagen disease involving the skin.

Diabetes—A condition of metabolism in which sugars and starches cannot be properly handled because of an inadequacy of insulin from the pancreas.

Diuresis—The act of producing urine.

DNA—(Desoxyribonucleic acid). A protein serving an essential function in the nucleus of cells.

Dysentery—A bloody diarrhea.

Dysmenorrhea—Painful menstruation.

Dyspepsia—Indigestion.

Dyspnea—Difficulty breathing.

Eclampsia—A toxic condition of pregnancy.

Eczema—A weeping, reddened, scaling dermatitis.

Elastic fiber—Connective tissue of the skin capable of contraction and expansion.

Encephalitis—An inflammation of the brain.

Endocarditis—An inflammation of the lining of the heart.

Endocrine glands—An organ which secretes hormones directly into the blood stream.

Endometriosis—Misplaced lining cells from the uterus.

Endometritis—Inflammation of the lining of the uterus.

Endothelial cells—The lining cells of all blood vessels and lymphatic vessels.

Enterohepatic circulation—The cycle of the taking up of bile from the small bowel and transporting it through the blood stream to the liver where it is secreted back into the bile for reabsorption from the small bowel.

Epidermis—The outer five layers of the skin, literally "over the skin".

Epididymitis—An inflammation of the epididymis, a small structure adjacent to the testes.

Erythroblastosis fetalis—A condition in infants of incompatibility of blood factors, specifically Rh factors.

Exudates—Material which oozes from blood vessels in response to infection or inflammation.

Fomentations—The application of heat with wet packs.

Fractures—Broken bones.

General adaptation syndrome—The stages of stress response by the body (alarm, followed by defense, and finally exhaustion).

Glycogenolysis—The process of making blood sugar for energy from the storage form of carbohydrate—glycogen.

Glycogen—The storage form of carbohydrate.

Herpes—A viral infection giving lesions on the lips, skin, and genital area.

Histamine—A powerful dilator of the capillaries.

Hubbard tank—A whirlpool tub.

Hyperpyrexia—Increased body temperature above what is normal.

Hypothermia—Below normal temperature.

Hypothyroidism—Below normal thyroid function.

Immune bodies—Antibodies.

Immune system—The body's system for producing antibodies.

Impacted feces—Hard and packed fecal material in the bowel requiring being broken up by the gloved finger.

Impetigo—An acute skin infection, usually in children, and usually caused by a streptococcus.

Isoniazid—An antituberculous drug.

Kaopectate—Kaolin (clay) and pectins (fiber from fruit). A preparation used for diarrhea, or nausea and vomiting.

Karyotype—A classification of chromosomes.

Keratitis—An inflammation of the eye.

Kernicterus—A condition of staining of the nuclei of the brain by bile pigments usually seen in severe erythroblastosis.

Kidney tubules—The tiniest tubes which transport urine and are responsible for maintaining the blood in a condition compatible with life.

Locomotion—Active movement of a whole organism.

Lymph—Interstitial fluid that has bathed the body tissues.

Lymphatic system—Collecting mechanisms primarily responsible for returning excess tissue fluid to the blood.

Lysins—Substances that break down structures such as blood cells or blood clots.

Macrophages—Large white blood cells that eat. Literally large feeding cells.

Mastitis—An inflammation of the breasts.

Mastoiditis—An inflammation of the mastoid sinuses, air filled cavities inside the temporal bone just behind the ear which communicate with the middle ear.

Melanin—The black pigment of the skin which imparts a tan color.

Menstruation—Normal uterine bleeding occuring monthly caused by the shedding of the endometrium.

Metabolism—The sum of the physical and chemical changes that occur in the body.

Motor nerves—The nerves that activate muscles and glands.

Muscular atrophy—A wasting muscle disease.

Muscular dystrophy—A wasting muscle disease.

Mutagens—Substances which cause mutations in the body. These mutations are always harmful.

Myositis—An inflammation of muscles.

Neuromuscular transmission—The sending of an impulse between nerves and muscles.

Neutrophils—A type of white blood cell which actively combats germs and other acute inflammatory producers.

Nightshades—A large botanical family including tomatoes, potatoes, eggplant, peppers, tobacco and many others.

Pacinian corpuscle—An organized nerve ending believed to be receptive to pressure.

Palpitation—The sensation that accompanies rapid heartbeat.

Pemphigus—A condition of skin characterized by generalized blister formation carrying a high mortality rate.

Perineal care—The hygiene of the external female genitalia.

Phagocytosis—Activity in which a cell takes solids into its cell by enfolding or formation of a "food cup". Literally the act of eating by cells.

Pharynx—The area back of the throat located between the mouth and the upper end of the esophagus.

Placebo—A substance given to "please" the patient, generally considered to be inactive.

Plague—A widespread contagious disease with a high death rate, specifically a disease characterized by high fever, restlessness, shock and coma.

Pleurisy—An inflammation of the pleura, the lining membrane of the chest and covering of the lungs.

Prenatal influences—Those influences brought to bear during pregnancy. Literally before birth.

Rete Pegs—Projections of the epidermis which anchor the outer layers of skin into the dermis.

Retroversion, uterine—A backward bending of the uterus. Forward bending is more usual.

Rosacea—A dermatitis characterized by papules and pustules.

Rubeola—Measles.

Sebaceous glands—Oil glands discharging their secretion into the hair follicle, producing sebum which keeps the skin lubricated.

Seminal vesicles—Tubular reservoirs which contain a fluid; a part of the male genitalia.

Shingles—A dermatitis occuring along a nerve route caused by the Herpes virus and characterized by blisters.

Shunt—A diversionary passage causing blood to flow from one passage to another.

Somnolence—Sleepiness.

Sudoresis—Sweating.

Sympathetic nervous system—The part of the nervous system having to do with "fight or flight".

Tetanus—Lockjaw.

Thoracic—Pertaining to the chest.

Thyroid gland—An endocrine gland located in the neck in front of the trachea.

Tic douloureux—A painful flashing, usually of a branch of the facial or mandibular nerve.

Urea—The chief nitrogenous product resulting from protein metabolism.

Uterus—The womb.

Uremia—The accumulation of urinary wastes in the blood because of kidney failure.

Ureters—The tubes which lead from the kidneys to the urinary bladder.

Uterine Atony—Lack of tone in the uterus occuring during labor.

Uterine retroversion—(see retroversion)

Vagina—The passageway for infant birth.

Vascular—Pertaining to vessels.

Vasoconstriction—Narrowing of blood vessels.

Vasodilator—A substance that dilates blood vessels.

Vasomotor—Having to do with the action of blood vessels.

Venule—A tiny vein.

White blood cells—Certain types of blood cells that constitute the defense system of the blood.

BIBLIOGRAPHY

1. Minnesota Medicine 54:973-979, December, 1971
2. White, Ellen G. Medical Ministry, Mountain View, California: Pacific Press Publishing Association, 1932, p. 83-84
3. White, Ellen G. The Ministry of Healing, Mountain View, California: Pacific Press Publishing Association, 1942, p. 128.
4. Unpublished Testimonies, January 8, 1892
5. Ibid.
6. White, Ellen G. Spiritual Gifts, Vol. 4, Battle Creek, Michigan: Review and Herald Publishing Association, 1864, p. 133
7. White, Ellen G. Counsels on Health, Mountain View, California: Pacific Press Publishing Association, 1923, p. 501
8. White, Ellen G. Selected Messages, Volume 2, Washington, D.C.: Review and Herald Publishing Association, 1958, p. 346
9. White, Ellen G. Spiritual Gifts, Volume 2, Battle Creek, Michigan: Review and Herald Publishing Association, 1864, p. 135
10. White, Ellen G. Testimonies to the Church, Volume 6, Mountain View, California: Pacific Press Publishing Association, 1948, p. 301
11. Journal of the American Medical Association 27:1330, December 26, 1896
12. British Journal of Physical Medicine 19:176-180, August, 1956
13. Physical Therapeutics 45:534-541, November, 1927
14. The Urologic and Cutaneous Review 42:258, 261. April, 1938
15. Medical Clinics of North America 33:1121-1130, July, 1949
16. Journal of the American Medical Association 89:502-506, August 13, 1927
17. Journal of the American Medical Association 230:1320-1321, December 2, 1974
18. Medical Times 104:88, November, 1976
19. Infection and Immunity 18:673-679, December, 1977
20. American Journal of Physiology 66:185-190, September 25, 1923
21. Medical Times 104:88-109, November, 1976
22. Physical Therapeutics 49:149-162, April, 1931
23. Medical Arts and Sciences 13:126-138, 1959
24. American Journal of Physiology 66:185-190, September 25, 1923
25. Physiological Abstracts 3:224, 1918
26. American Journal of Physiology 66:187, September 25, 1923
27. Medical Arts and Sciences 13:126-139, 1959
28. American Journal of Medical Science 193:470, April, 1937
29. Science News 111:328, May 21, 1977
30. American Journal of Physiology 66:185, September 25, 1923
31. The Lancet 1:263, February 7, 1976
32. Medical World News, April 4, 1969, p. 37
33. American Journal of Medical Sciences 201:115, January, 1941
34. Science News 110:55, July 24, 1976
35. Science News 107:237, April 12, 1975
36. Medical Counterpoint, August, 1973, p. 5
37. New England Journal of Medicine 298:607-612, March 16, 1978
38. Hospital Practice, 11:56, May, 1976
39. Archives of Physical Therapy 19:143, March, 1938
40. Medical Arts and Sciences 13:127, 1959
41. White, Ellen G, Education, Mountain View, California: Pacific Press Publishing Association, 1903, p. 198, 199
42. The Lancet 1:1229, June 2, 1973
43. Journal of the American Medical Association 106:1158, April 4, 1936
44. Kellogg, J. H. Rational Hydrotherapy. Philadelphia: F. A. Davis Co. 1903, p. 79-80
45. Israeli Journal of Medical Science 12:759-764, 1976
46. Journal of the American Medical Association 237(16):1691, April 19, 1977
47. Israeli Journal of Medical Science 12:759-764, 1976
48. Southern Medical Journal 73(8):963-964, August, 1980
49. The Lancet 277:178, July 23, 1977
50. American Journal of Physiology 70:412-429, October, 1924
51. American Journal of Syphilis 11:337-397, July, 1927
52. Physiotherapy 62(3):86, March, 1976
53. Science News 110:55, July 24, 1976
54. Infection and Immunity 18:673-679, December, 1977
55. Physical Therapeutics 45:354-541, November, 1927
56. Health Reformer 7(6):187, June, 1872
57. Clinical Science 36:419-426, 1969
58. Selye, Hans, Stress, Montreal, Canada: Acta, Inc. Medical Publishers
59. Physician and Sportmedicine, November, 1976, p 67-69
60. Physical Therapy Review 39:598-599, September, 1959
61. Physical Therapy Review 39:598, September, 1959
62. Journal of the American Medical Association 40.1081, April 18, 1903
63. Medical Arts and Sciences 13(3):126-138, 1959
64. Bulletin of the Battle Creek Sanitarium and Hospital Clinic 23:127-152, August, 1928
65. Archives of Physical Therapy 19:135, March, 1938
66. Archives of Physical Therapy 19:138, March, 1938
67. Archives of Physical Therapy 19:135-143, March, 1938
68. Medical Arts and Sciences 13:126-138, 1959
69. Bulletin of the Battle Creek Sanitarium and Hospital Clinic 23:129-152, August, 1928
70. Selye, Hans. Stress. Acta, Inc. Medical Publishers, Montreal, Canada 1950, page 651
71. Cancer Research 3:464-470, July, 1943
72. Rothweller and White. Art and Science of Nursing. 4th Edition. Philadelphia, F. A. Davis Co. 1952
73. Journal of the American Medical Association 157:1189, April 2, 1955
74. Journal of the American Medical Association 15:72, July 12, 1890
75. Journal of the American Medical Association 27:1330-34, December 26, 1896
76. Medical Arts and Sciences 13(3):126-138, 1959
77. Physical Therapeutics 45:534-541, November, 1927
78. Journal of Aviation Medicine 20:179-185, June, 1949
79. Annals of Chemical Research 8:266-271, 1976
80. Journal of Small Animal Practice 12:179-184, March, 1971

81. The Lancet 1:519-520, March 11, 1978
82. Guy's Hospital Reports 11:225-262, 1969
83. Science News 114:285, October 21, 1978
84. Journal of the American Medical Association 219:1486, March 13, 1972
85. Medical Letter on Drugs and Therapeutics 12:3-4, January 9, 1970
86. Urologic and Cutaneous Review 42:258, 261, April, 1938
87. White, Ellen G. Selected Messages, Volume 2, Mountain View, California: Pacific Press Publishing Association, p. 290
88. Clinical Electroencephalography 11(1):122-127, January, 1980
89. Medical Bulletin of the Veteran's Administration 7:1083-1085, November, 1931
90. Archives of Physical Medicine 50:597-603, 608, October 1969
91. Journal of the American Physical Therapy Association 44:713-717, August, 1964
92. Archives of Physical Medicine 50:597-603, 608, October, 1969
93. British Journal of Haematology 16:409-11, April 1969
94. Fever Therapy. New York; Paul B. Hoebner, Inc. 1937
95. Clinical Pediatrics 15:776, 1976
96. Medical Record, February 27, 1904, p. 326-330
97. Journal of Advanced Therapeutics 21:20-26, 1903
98. Illinois Medical Journal April, 1911, p. 447-451
99. Archives of Medical Hydrology 7:197-200, May, 1929
100. Munchener Medizinische Wochenschrift 98:360-362, March 16, 1956
101. Zeitschrift fur die gesamte Physikalische Therapie 37:161-164, August 23, 1929
102. British Journal of Physical Medicine, March, 1930, p. 250, 251
103. Journal of the American Medical Association 5:36, June 15, 1901
104. Journal of the American Medical Association 35:232, July 28, 1900
105. Finnerty, Gertrude. Hydrotherapy. New York: Frederick Ungar Pub. Co. 1960
106. Archives of Ophthalmology 32:296, October, 1944
107. Archives of Physical Therapy 18:199-205, April, 1937
108. Abbott, George K. Physical Therapy in Nursing Care. Takoma Park, Washington D.C. Review and Herald Publishing House, 1945, p. 141
109. Medical Journal of Malaysia 30(3):221-223 March, 1976
110. Physical Therapy 50:193-194, February, 1970
111. Indian Medical Record, June, 1930, p. 92A
112. Journal of the American Medical Association 107:230, July 18, 1936
113. Medical Record August 25, 1916, p. 367, 368
114. Journal of the American Medical Association 243(4):370, January 25, 1980

115. American Journal of Physiology 70:412, October, 1924
116. American Journal of Clinical Nutrition 25:231, February, 1972
117. Medical Arts and Sciences 13(3):126, 1959
118. Cancer 34:122-129, 1974
119. American Journal of Roentgenology 33:75-87, 1935
120. Cancer Research 3:2568-2578, November, 1973
121. Annals of the Royal College of Surgeons of England 54:72, February, 1974
122. Annals of the Royal College of Surgeons of England 54:72, February, 1974
123. Medical World News, May 29, 1978
124. Medical World News, November 15, 1975, p. 57
125. Journal of the American Medical Association 236(25):2845, December 20, 1976
126. International Journal of Biometerology 13:183-187, October, 1969
127. Journal of Clinical Pathology 29:1-10, 1976
128. Bulletin of the Calcutta School of Tropical Medicine 12:20-21, January, 1964
129. Journal of the American Medical Association 65:1882, May 29, 1915
130. Journal of the American Medical Association 65:288, July 17, 1915
131. Journal of the American Medical Association 109(2):111, July 10, 1937
132. Journal of the American Medical Association 110(23):1958, June 4, 1938
133. Medical World News, September 17, 1979
134. Journal of the American Medical Association 37:1075, October 19, 1901
135. Archives of Physical Medicine 50:597, October, 1969
136. Archives of Physical Medicine and Rehabilitation 50:603-608, October, 1969
137. Journal of the American Medical Association 40:129, January 10, 1903
138. Medical World News, May 16, 1977 p. 20
139. Proceedings of the Society for Experimental Biology and Medicine 26:287-288, January, 1929
140. Illinois Medical Journal, July 1941, p. 31-32
141. Journal of the American Medical Association 216(2):1926, June 21, 1971
142. Journal of the American Medical Association 36:1304, May 11, 1901
143. Archives of Pediatrics, May, 1908, p. 358-367
144. Medical Bulletin of the Veterans Administration 7:1083-1085, November, 1931
145. Medical Record, August 26, 1916, p. 367-368
146. Physical Therapeutics 47:89-91, February, 1929
147. Journal of the American Medical Association 27:1330, December 26, 1896
148. Annals of Internal Medicine 11:160, March, 1938
149. Journal of the American Medical Association 109:904, September 11, 1937

150. Klinische Wochenschrift 7:1899-1901, September 30, 1928
151. Canadian Medical Association Journal 75:388-394, September 1, 1956
152. Archives of Ophthalmology 19:769, May, 1938
153. British Journal of Venereal Disease 47:293-4, 1971
154. Munchener Medizinische Wochenschrift 92:224-228, May 12, 1950
155. Indian Medical Record 50:97A-102A, June, 1930
156. Journal of the American Medical Association 40:129, January 10, 1903
157. Journal of the American Medical Association 34:675, March 17, 1900
158. Transactions of the American Hospital Association 32:501, 1930
159. Transactions of the American Hospital Association 32:500-506, 1930
160. Journal of the American Medical Association 61:522, August 16, 1913
161. Maryland Medical Journal, April, 1905, p. 129-132
162. Archives of Physical Medicine 39:281-285, February, 1927
163. American Journal of Medical Sciences 107:502-515, 1894
164. Proceedings of the Society for Experimental Biology and Medicine 31:87-91, October, 1933
165. The Physician and Sportsmedicine 8(12):25, December, 1980
166. Klinische Wochenschrift 50:332-444, March 15, 1972
167. British Journal of Physical Medicine 19:176-180, August, 1956
168. Der Hautarzt 4:565-567, December, 1953
169. Quarterly Journal of Medicine 1:387-400, July, 1932
170. Pediatrics 46(3):445, September, 1970
171. Quarterly Journal of Studies on Alcohol 3:31-33, June, 1942
172. Buffalo Medical Journal, September, 1903
173. Journal of the American Medical Association 111(11):1017, September 10, 1938
174. Edinburgh Medical Journal, October, 1912, p. 319
175. Journal of the American Medical Association 219(12):1643, March 20, 1972
176. Valsalva 4:202-213, April, 1929
177. Journal of the American Medical Association 23:236-240, August 11, 1894
178. Physical Therapy Reviews 40:93-99, February, 1960
179. Ostrom, Kurre W. Massage and the Original Swedish Movements. Philadelphia: P. Blakeston Son and Co. 1906
180. Maryland Medical Journal, April 1905, p. 29-32
181. British Medical Journal, August 26, 1972
182. Cooney, David O. Activated Charcoal. New York: Marcel Dekker, Inc. 1980, p. 47
183. Acta Pharmacologica et Toxicologica 4:275, 1948
184. Journal of the American Medical Association 64:1882, May 29, 1915

185. Cooney, David O. Activated Charcoal. New York: Marcel Dekker, Inc. 1980 p. 33
186. Journal of the American Medical Association 210(10):1846, December 8, 1969
187. Bulletin de la Society de Chime Biologique 27:513-518, October-December, 1945
188. Journal of Animal Science 34:322-325, February, 1972
189. Cooney, David O. Activated Charcoal. New York: Marcel Dekker, Inc. 1980 p. 63
190. Clinical Toxicology 3(1):1-4, March, 1970
191. Annals of Emergency Medicine 9:11, November, 1980
192. AMA Archives of Industrial Health 18:511-520, December, 1958
193. Archives of Environmental Health 1:512, December, 1960
194. Journal of the American Medical Association 240(7):684, August 18, 1978
195. Comptes rendus Hebdomadaires des Seance de 1-Academie des Sciences 187:959-961, November 19, 1928
196. Toxicology and Applied Pharmacology 26:103-108, September, 1973
197. Journal of the American Medical Association 209(12):1821, September 22, 1969
198. Journal of the American Medical Association 237(17):1840, April 25, 1976
199. Journal of the American Medical Association 54:331, December 7, 1910
200. Patient Care, October 30, 1977 p. 152
201. Eye, Ear, Nose and Throat Monthly 47:652-655, December, 1968
202. Journal of the American Geriatrics Society 12:500-502, May, 1964
203. Journal of the American Medical Association 64:1671, 1915
204. Chirurg 19:191, April, 1948
205. Quarterly Journal of Pharmacology 1:334-337, July-September, 1928
206. Cooney, David O. Activated Charcoal. New York: Marcel Dekker, Inc. 1980, p. 123
207. Ibid, p. 131
208. Ibid, p. 133
209. White, Ellen G. Selected Messages, Volume Two, Washington, D.C. Review and Herald Publishing Association, 1958 p. 294
210. Nature 184(Suppl 15):1165-6, October 10, 1959
211. Medical World News, February 17, 1967
212. Cooney, David O. Activated Charcoal. New York: Marcel Dekker, Inc. 1980
213. The Lancet 1:1301, 1974
214. Annals of Internal Medicine 93:446-449, 1980

215. British Medical Journal 2:1465, November 25, 1978
216. Medical Tribune, April 12, 1978, p. 2
217. Surgery, Gynecology, and Obstetrics 96:873-878, 1930
218. White, Ellen G. K-100-1903
219. Dextreit, Raymond, Our Earth, Our Cure, Brooklyn, New York: Swan House Publishing Company, 1974
220. Chemical and Pharmaceutical Bulletin 17(11):2193-2197, November, 1969
221. Journal of Scientific and Industrial Research. Section C: Biological Sciences 20C:292-295, October, 1961
222. Journal of Scientific and Industrial Research. Section C: Biological Sciences 5(2):2461, August, 1946
223. Chinese Medical Journal 93(2):123-126, 1980
224. The Lancet 2:1491, December 29, 1973
225. Journal of the American Veterinary Association 102:109-111, February, 1943
226. Cancer Research 20:431-434, May, 1960
227. Nature 216:83-84, October 7, 1967
228. Watanabe, Taoashi. Garlic Therapy. Tokyo: Japan Publications, 1974
229. American Journal of Tropical Medicine and Hygeine 18:920-923, November, 1969
230. International Journal of Dermatology 19(5):285-287, June, 1980
231. Journal of Scientific and Industrial Research 5(2):2461, August, 1946
232. Food Research 5:503-507, September-October, 1940
233. Chinese Medical Journal 93(2):123-126, February, 1980
234. Indian Journal of Experimental Biology 15:466-468, June, 1977
235. Medical Record 153:249-251, April, 1941
236. Journal of the Indian Medical Association 39:517-520, November, 1962
237. Archivum Immunologiae et Therapiae Experimentalis 12:96-105, 1964
238. Acta Microbiologica Polonica, Series B 5(22):51-62
239. Chemistry December, 1977
240. Advances in Enzymology and Related Subjects 11:377-400, 1951
241. Journal of the Royal Egyptian Medical Association, January-February, 1946, p. 90-100
242. The Antiseptic 43:631-632, October, 1946
243. Journal of the Indian Medical Association 22:14-15, October, 1952
244. Journal of the American Chemical Society 66:1950-1, 1944

245. Review of Gastroenterology 2:22, January-February, 1944
246. Zentralblatt fur Gynakelogie 54:1690-1692, July 5, 1930
247. Japanese Journal of Pharmacy 19:1-4, March, 1969
248. Buffalo Evening News, September 5, 1978
249. Indian Heart Journal 30(1):47, 1978
250. Atherosclerosis 29:125-129, February, 1978
251. Journal of Nutrition 110(5):731-6, May, 1980
252. Medical Record 153:249-251, April, 1941
253. New Orleans Medical and Surgical Journal, August, 1911, p. 131, 132
254. Advances in Prostaglandin and Thromboxane Research 6:309-312, 1980
255. Prostaglandins and Medicine 2:413-424, 1979
256. Atherosclerosis 30:355-360, August, 1978
257. Canadian Medical Association Journal 100:626, April 5, 1969
258. British Medical Journal 3:351, August 10, 1968
259. Indian Journal of Medical Research 54:48-53, January, 1966
260. Journal of Nutrition 110:931-936, 1980
261. Science 174:1343, December, 1971
262. Illinois Medical Journal, July, 1941 p. 31-32
263. Physical Therapy 52:273 8, March, 1972
264. Handbook of the Medical Sciences 4:40, 1914
265. Atherosclerosis 21:15-19, 1975
266. The Lancet 2:1491, December 29, 1973
267. Kordel, LeLord. Natural Folk Remedies. New York:G. P. Putnam's Sons, 1974
268. American Journal of Clinical Nutrition 28(7):684-5, July, 1975
269. The Lancet 1:145, January 19, 1980
270. The Lancet 2:1491, December 29, 1973
271. Annals of Internal Medicine 93:446-449, 1980
272. Abbott, George Knapp. Physical Therapy in Nursing Care Takoma Park: Washington, D.C.: Review and Herald Publishing Association, 1945 p. 64-65
273. Cooney, David O. Activated Charcoal. New York: Marcel Dekker, Inc. 1980 p. 4
274. New England Journal of Medicine 301:216, July 26, 1979
275. Science News 112:343, November 19, 1977

INDEX

Uchee Pines Lifestyle Center

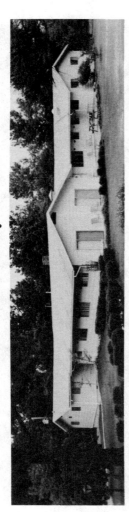

Your body knows naturally what it needs to stay healthy. And it tries to tell you...but have you been listening?

Most of us eat and drink too much, eat the wrong kinds of foods, drink beverages that are hard on body systems, exercise frantically, and them feel worse rather than better. We can't relax when we "rest". We ignore the natural rhythms and requests of our bodies — and we get sick as a result.

But we can eat healthful foods prepared in healthful ways, drink the refreshing drinks nature provides, exercise through purposeful labor that is more beneficial than frantic "recreation". We can rest in natural tranquility. If we learn these simple skills, we stay healthy — really healthy...

Or we get well if we're sick.

Anvwodi (ah-niv-wo-di), the Cherokee word for "get well place", is the Lifestyle Center at Uchee Pines. Here you learn to keep yourself in good health through use of nature's most powerful "drugs": pure air, sunlight, temperance, rest, spiritual support, exercise, proper diet, and that beneficial liquid — water. You become whole again while enjoying the peace and serenity of two hundred acres of pine and oak woodland.

You'll have your own program of specially prescribed conditioning treatments. When you arrive you'll be given a physical examination and a laboratory analysis.

Based on the results and a comprehensive medical interview, you'll be given a program of rest, activity, diet, demonstrations, lectures, and natural therapy to bring you toward the peak of good health.

And of course, your physical and medical needs will be constantly monitored.

You'll eat fresh and delicious meals of homegrown fruits and vegetables, homemade cereals and natural breads — and learn how to prepare such healthful meals for yourself.

You'll breathe in life-restoring, pollution-free air and drink up Southern sunlight while gardening, hiking, chopping wood, or tending the orchard — the kind of labor that feels good because you're putting your muscles to healthy use.

You'll learn to use water to greatest advantage — to drink, to stimulate, to soothe.

You may choose to seek the warmth of family worship. You can elect this experience at Anvwodi. And if you wish, one of our chaplains will listen and discuss your spiritual concerns.

When you go home, how will you feel? If you continue the good, healthful habits you've learned at Uchee Pines, you'll continue to feel as if you were still in the beautiful Alabama woodland, living a clean, simple, invigorating life.

What we're offering you is a lifetime of better living...as the Creator intended.

☐ YES, please send me more information about how I can condition myself for better living at Uchee Pines.

☐ I'd like to talk with someone about the health conditioning program. My number ( )

Name _____

Address _____

City _____ ST _____ Zip _____

Uchee Pines Lifestyle Center
30 Uchee Pines Rd., #75
Seale, AL 36875
Phone: (334) 855-4764